WATER BIRTH

A Midwife's Perspective

Susanna Napierala

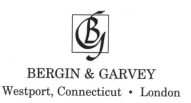

BERGIN & GARVEY

Westport, Connecticut • London

While the advice and information in this book are believed to be true and accurate at the date of going to press, neither the author nor the publisher can accept any legal responsibility for any errors or omissions that may be made. The publisher makes no warranty, express or implied, with respect to the material contained herein. Readers are encouraged to confirm the information in this volume with other sources.

Library of Congress Cataloging-in-Publication Data

Napierala, Susanna.
    Water birth : a midwife's perspective / Susanna Napierala.
      p. cm.
    Includes bibliographical references and index.
    ISBN 0–89789–285–2 (pb)
    1. Underwater childbirth. I. Title.
RG663.N37   1994
618.4—dc20   93–49703

British Library Cataloguing in Publication Data is available.

Library of Congress Catalog Card Number: 93–49703
ISBN: 0–89789–285–2 (pbk.)

First published in 1994

Bergin & Garvey, 88 Post Road West, Westport, CT 06881
An imprint of Greenwood Publishing Group, Inc.

Printed in the United States of America

The paper used in this book complies with the
Permanent Paper Standard issued by the National
Information Standards Organization (Z39.48–1984).

10 9 8 7 6 5

Every reasonable effort has been made to trace the owners of copyright materials in this book, but in some instances this has proven impossible. The author and publisher will be glad to receive information leading to more complete acknowledgments in subsequent printings of the book and in the meantime extend their apologies for any omissions.

This book is dedicated to my son, Nathaniel Napierala, who has ventured forth with me during his ten years, helping me research this book, understanding when I have had to write, and totally loving me.

Also to my husband, Jeff Cox, who has held my hand and advised me during the writing of this book, and given me his loving support and understanding.

And to my parents, Florence and Henry Napierala, for loving me and giving me a good start.

CONTENTS

ACKNOWLEDGMENTS

I would like to give special thanks to Sonoma State University. The English Department and Women's Studies Department have given me much support during the writing of this book. To Professors David Bromidge, Gerald Haslam, Larry Levinger, and Cindy Stearns, thank you.

I would also like to thank my friends and associates for their encouragement in researching and writing this book: Rick Genstil, Marty Wagner, Dr. Mary Davenport, Katy O'Leary CNM, Phyllis Glickstein P.A., the RV *Heraclitus* and her crew, my Russian and Ukranian friends, and all those who have encouraged me and supported me in this endeavor.

Special thanks to Dr. Sharon Olson for sharing her medical expertise, to Jeff René for his contribution for the birthing tank section, and to Margaret Ewing for her translation of "A Water Birth in 1805."

INTRODUCTION

In 1981 only a few babies had been born under water. During that year, I was teaching a childbirth class at my home in Glen Ellen, California. We were fortunate to catch a television program showing the pioneering birthing techniques of Igor Charkowsky, a Russian midwife and swimming instructor, who had been experimenting since the early 1960s with water births. My class watched fascinated as women gave birth peacefully into the water. The feeling in the class was: "That's for me!"

Inspired by the television program, two of my students, Rennie and Larry, asked me to help them with a water birth and to serve as their midwife. When I agreed, Larry began building their birthing tank. We gave each other assignments to research the various aspects of underwater births. I wanted some technical medical questions answered before I could feel safe venturing down paths that had barely been beaten. Most of all, I inquired, doesn't the baby have to breathe? What about blood loss? Infections? In my desire to find out what initiates the first breath of the newborn, I soon found myself poring over medical texts and research papers at Stanford's medical library. The medical scientists seemed to have their theories, but none of them convinced me that they really knew the physiological mechanism. I was to find this out myself.

As a midwife, more than once I've encountered the situation where the labor just isn't progressing. When this happens, hours can pass in difficult labor. One technique I've always used to help the woman in difficult labor relax is to have her get into a tub of warm water. I've seen 2 to 3 centimeters of dilation occur almost immediately after immersion as this gentle medium works its effects on the woman's laboring body. Comparable progress usually takes hours in the absence of the water bath. I've also seen the Leboyer water baths relax newborns, their tight fists unfolding like flowers and their faces, strained from birth, becoming serene. Over the years, I had never given water's effects too much thought; it was simply one of several tricks midwives use to help mothers give birth.

On a beautiful day in February, Rennie's baby decided to make her debut. Watching with amazement, I was delighted to see how well the water helped Rennie go through transition. Trying to be objective about the labor wasn't easy, for the buoyancy and warmth of the water seemed to be just the perfect medium for relaxation. When the baby's head started to appear, my brain said, "Well, you've really done it this time. You must be crazy!" Fortunately, that thought lasted only a second, and then my intuition told me, "Trust. You know this has been done before, you've researched this."

And so it was. The baby slowly and gently emerged from her mother's womb into the water. When she emerged as far as her chest, she opened her eyes and looked into her father's. There was seemingly a sense of recognition. Then she slowly closed her eyes, giving the appearance that she didn't know she had been born. She seemed to be sleeping. One of Rennie's friends who was present remarked on the baby's serenity.

Robin (as the newborn was called) was born slowly and peacefully into the water. Her vital signs, such as heartbeat, muscle tone, and pulsation of the umbilical cord, were working strongly. Robin remained under water a total of eleven minutes. While everything went well in her case, I no longer advise or condone leaving newborns underwater for such an extended period of time. At this birth we were following the examples of the few water births that had occurred in the United States. Zero to two minutes is a sufficient amount of time for the stress to leave the baby; no marathons are needed.

With Robin's birth my work as a birth attendant underwent a great change. Never before in the four hundred births I had previously attended had I seen a baby born so gently and serenely. Nor had I witnessed the freedom of movement, with such little energy expended, as Rennie had enjoyed in the water.

As more parents asked for my support in attempting water births, my confidence and trust in the method grew. I recognized that this method could free women to labor more efficiently. Therefore, I began to research this information so that water would be accessible to more women and practitioners.

In the summer of 1982, I was invited to speak at the first International Underwater Birth Conference in Tutukaka, New Zealand. At this meeting physicians, midwives, and psychologists from all over the world gathered to discuss and learn about the benefits of water birthing for the mother and baby. I was particularly excited about the information that world champion breath-hold diver Jacques Mayol brought. His research into reduced rates of oxygen consumption while under water confirmed my own research and observations. I also met a Maori woman who told me that her people customarily gave birth in the warm springs on the island.

The conference was held in a small fishing village on the North Island of New Zealand, and was led by a small, intimate group of highly skilled professionals, who in their dedication to giving credibility to water births, shared much information and support. Information necessary for the safety of the mother and baby that had formerly been accessible only in the USSR and France was now available to the rest of the world. When I returned to the United States, I was brimming with confidence that water births are indeed beneficial for the mother and baby, and that many parents and professionals in other parts of the world agreed.

Little did I know how my confidence would be tested. The year 1984 brought my greatest personal experience in the realm of water births—the birth of my son Nathaniel. Instead of a little crib in the nursery, I set up a jacuzzi spa in the living room. I labored both in and out of the water. The water made a remarkable difference for me. Most importantly, in the water I was able to relax and dilate very easily and quickly—so quickly, in fact, that five minutes after my bag of waters broke at 5 centimeters, I felt the urge to push. Sure enough, my son was coming through, and there was no stopping him. Only thirty minutes elapsed from the time I reached 5 centimeters to the birth of Nathaniel. It should have taken at least another seven hours. What my heart and mind knew all along, my body and soul were finally able to discover. Yes, water does make a difference.

Both my research work and my own personal experience of birthing my son showed me the importance of letting go, a process aided immeasurably by giving birth in water.

In 1985 the Conscious Birthing Circle, a group of professionals consisting of physicians, midwives, psychologists, and psychics, was formed in San Francisco. Our main purpose was to research water births and perinatal psychology. Several members of the core group had visited Igor Charkowsky in the USSR. and found that it was difficult to see him in as much as his work was not sanctioned by his government. Nonetheless, it was worth the risk.

The year 1986 found Nathaniel and me hopping planes, boats, and trains, visiting various water birth centers in Europe as well as Charkowsky in Moscow. First, I traveled to Denmark where I visited a friend, keeping in mind the people in Europe with whom I had made contact through the birthing circle. Nathaniel and I took the train from

Copenhagen to Brussels, and then went on to a small hospital outside of Waterloo. I telephoned Dr. Serge Wesel, the hospital's director of obstetrics, who promptly came to the train station to drive me to the small country hospital. I was greeted by the *sage femmes* (midwives) who demonstrated their stool-like birthing chairs. They showed me the room where women could labor in a tub of warm water and birth on a bed close by. From there we traveled by train to a town by the sea, Oostende. People chuckled at two-year-old Nathaniel, as he pushed a wheeled suitcase as big as he was down the corridors of the train stations. In Oostende we visited Dr. Herman Ponnett, an obstetrician at a local hospital where a plexiglass tank is used to give birth in the water.

Then we went on to Paris by train. I loved the French countryside and thought of all the poems that had been written about the area. From Paris we went to London. A lecture was scheduled for me to speak about my work with women laboring and giving birth in water. There I met with Dr. Michel Odent, exchanging many ideas.

When I returned to Denmark, I realized that it was time to do more research. Most of all, I wanted to work with the pioneer of water births himself, Igor Charkowsky.

Arriving in the country that had so long been thought of as enemy territory brought back many childhood fears. Visions of Nikita Khrushchev beating his shoe on the table at the United Nations came into my mind as I went through the tight security channels. These fears were dispelled as soon as I met Charkowsky and the Russian midwives all of whom greeted me with broken English, hugs, and smiles.

Soon, they whisked me off through the gleaming, marble metro (Moscow's subway) to private homes. There I saw water babies, just a few months old, diving and swimming in the water. Other homes contained plexiglass tanks with women laboring in them. Some of these women were smiling; others appeared to be in meditation. Beautiful babies were born under water and were immediately taught to swim. I left Moscow having learned a great deal but also knowing that I needed more information.

In 1987 I returned to work with Charkowsky near Yalta, Crimea, in the Black Sea. We camped by the water's edge. Here rather than white sandy beaches, we had to live with hard rocks and a lack of facilities. I washed my hair in the sea and cooked in a big cast iron pot over the scraps of wood we gathered. Frequently, submarines would surface, displaying their hammer and sickles, ever reminding me of where I was.

When I arrived, two pregnant women were waiting to give birth in the sea. They and their partners prepared daily for birth through meditation and swimming. I watched in amazement as other babies, not yet able to walk, bobbed up and down in the sea, while dolphins swam by. It was like a fairy tale.

It was here that I saw Charkowsky in his true element. Since he spoke no English, he worked with an interpreter. Eventually, however, there was little need for interpretation. We worked well together, using hand motions when we needed to communicate. I watched him dunking young infants, propelling them through the water to their mothers. I found him to be a highly skilled midwife and swimming instructor. He is also able to work with kinds of energies that we are just discovering— or rediscovering. I actually saw him turn a breech baby by moving these energies with his hands. Here were tools that I needed—tools that a midwife doesn't find in an obstetric text. I returned to the states wondering how I was going to convey this discovery to the childbirth world.

My friends and colleagues kept encouraging me to write a book, reminding me of the lack of information available from a professional perspective. Pregnant couples from other states and countries kept calling me for more information on how and what to do to have a water birth. I feel compelled to share my experience and research.

My hope is that with some basic information, people will be able to make an educated decision as to whether or not homebirths and water births are appropriate for them. I know from personal experience that both mother and baby can safely enjoy the beauty and tranquility of the water. While I may know it, however, the decision is always the parents'.

This book is intended for prospective parents as well as for the prenatal caregiver and birth attendant—ideally, the same person. Traditionally, throughout the ages the midwife has handed down her knowledge and art to others. That is part of being a midwife and how the lineage has been kept. Accordingly, in this book I've included guidelines developed through my own practical experiences.

Working toward global peace and nonviolence is a major part of my commitment to midwifery and to life. Throughout the years I have accepted the basic premise that violence begets violence. As we well know, the newborn is a highly developed sensory being at birth. I hope the baby's first impressions will be not of harshness and segregation, but of security and gentleness. Without exception I have experienced this feeling of gentleness through underwater births. I am also commited to women and to parents, specifically to the notion that they should have the freedom of choice to give birth wherever, however, and with whomever they feel comfortable.

Many people, both laypersons and experts, believe that childbirth can affect the baby at birth and for the rest of his or her life. My hope is that people can be helped to come into the world in a loving, gentle manner and that this experience will be the first imprint on a new and trusting soul. Every new person should be greeted with love and respect at birth. Indeed, this is our inherent birthright.

This book is the product of thirteen years of research and five hundred homebirths, sixty-five of them water births. Based on my extensive studies and personal experience, I feel very confident that water is a safe alternative to drugs and other forms of intervention that are causing the United States to have some of the highest rates of infant mortality and caesarean sections in the industrialized world. A tank of warm water should be installed in every hospital as a means of helping women to relax, thus preventing complications for both mother and baby. Women intuitively know how to give birth, and water empowers them to do so.

For many years women in the United States have been concentrating their efforts on informing both men and women about women's reproductive rights. However, in their fight for their reproductive rights, women have left an important and basic issue by the wayside: freedom of choice during pregnancy and childbirth; the right to have a nonmedicalized labor and delivery, free from unnecessary intervention and technology. Giving birth is a function that women inherently know how to perform, if left alone for nature to take its course. Women also need to take responsibility for themselves and not be afraid of their bodies. Their bodies were made to give birth for the continuation of the species. There is no mystery about it. If women educate themselves about birth and trust in their bodies, they will suffer fewer complications for both themselves and their babies.

It is these thoughts that motivated this book. I do not believe that laboring or birthing in the water is for everyone, but it is an option that should be available to any person who desires it. Through this book I hope to share my knowledge and beautiful experiences with water, which may help others avail themselves of that choice.

Warning: The instructions and advice presented in this book are in no way intended as a substitute for medical counseling. The information contained in this book may not be suitable for everyone, and may be more applicable to certain persons and certain conditions than others. In an effort to reduce any risk of harm in your specific case, you should consult with your doctor or midwife before beginning or continuing to work with any of the suggestions described in this book. Water births are not suitable for everyone.

I

THE NATURE OF WATER

Water is the cradle of life here on earth. Life originated in the ocean more than three billion years ago. Somewhere in the warm seas, the first primitive creatures were formed, increased in number, developed.

Igor Charkowsky, quoted in Erik Sidenbladh, *Water Babies*

WATER

Water is our mother. Evolutionists believe we emerged from her cradle, the sea, millions of years ago. Our first nine months of existence took place in the waters of the womb. Perhaps this is why people feel such an affinity for water. The sound of the ocean's waves are echoes of the blood rushing through the placenta, the familiar sounds of the first few months of our existence.

Water's qualities are innumerable. It is able to hold hot and cold, to conduct and to transfer. Absorption of temperatures is just one of its amazing qualities.

Water is common in everything—plants, animals, and humans. It is the universal element that ties together all three of these classifications of life—it is itself a living being. Water is the most precious of our natural resources. It maintains life.

Theodor Schwenk, founder of the Institute for Flow Sciences in Herrischried, Germany, studied water as a lifegiving element and wrote of it in his two books, *Sensitive Chaos* (1976) and *Water: The Element of Life* (1989). He reminds us that 70 percent of the earth is covered with water. Schwenk described water as having these properties:

- Renouncing any form of its own, it becomes the creative matrix for form in everything else.
- Renouncing any life of its own, it becomes the primal substance of all life.
- Renouncing material fixity, it becomes the implementer of material change.
- Renouncing any rhythm of its own, it becomes the progenitor of rhythm elsewhere.

Schwenk continues with his description of water as keeping a balance:

- Between life and death.
- Between gravity and levity.
- Between light and darkness: giving rise to the rainbow when interacting with water.
- Between base and acid: mediating all chemical change.
- Between stillness and movement, whose interplay forms the basis for every rhythm and every pulsebeat.

WATER AND HUMANS

Every cell of our body contains mostly water. A newborn's body is made up of over 90 percent water, while an adult's is about 60 percent. Water assists in one of our most important bodily functions—breaking down food and converting it into fuel. From there it aids in breaking it down for the flushing process of elimination. It is important for the entire metabolic process, including regulation of the body temperature. The brain itself is in a buoyant state, floating in a fluid at the top of the body, less susceptible to the pull of gravity.

Water also affects the skin, our largest organ. In our skin are millions of nerves that are sensitive to heat, cold, and pain. These receptors give feedback to our central nervous system. If the skin goes through a temperature change, such as being in water, these nerves inform the body how to react. For instance, when warm water is applied to a sore muscle, the blood vessels dilate, bringing more blood to the area where the heat is. Muscles and tendons will relax.

Throughout time water has been revered for its spiritual, healing, and lifegiving qualities. It was not long ago in history that we had to haul water for our daily purposes. It was a precious commodity. Now with our modern-day systems, all we need to do is turn on the tap and there it is. When water becomes unavailable in our daily lives, it is then that we become aware of just how precious that commodity is. Usually, however, water is something we take for granted. We have lost our respect for water, and in a sense, we have lost a part of our heritage that has enriched our lives.

WATER AND RELIGION

Water has been a source of rituals, myths, and legends for centuries, and since the beginning of time, it has been thought of as a feminine element, being the beginning of the first sign of life. The earliest culture-bearers, preceding the male gods, were the feminine gods from the sea in fish form. The fish has been a symbol of fertility in many cultures.

From the Assyrian pantheon is the goddess An Zu who is linked with the goddess Ishtar. Both symbolize the primordial water. Artemis is the Greek goddess of the waters of the land—the lakes, marshes, and streams. She is often depicted with water hair and streams of life flowing down from her waist.

In Sumerian, the word *Mari* means both womb and sea. Aphrodite-Mari was known at the Hierapolis as the mother to us all, born of the sea, and she is said to have produced all from the watery fluid. In her Greek form, she stands on a dolphin, which was believed to be a fish by the Greeks. In Sanskrit, the goddess of love means "she who has a fish as her emblem." Many other goddesses have been identified with water and with resurrection: the Virgin Mary, Kali, Themis, Atargatis, and Tiamat.

Water has been a central element for many cultures and religions. The ancient Peruvians, for example, considered themselves the children of water. They set up altars near streams and lakes and held water to be sacred. The high priests would dive into the deepest fountains or pools with their offerings to the goddess of water. Similarly, the Celts worshiped wells. Their goddess Aerfon was also called Dyfridwy, translated as "water of divinity." For their part, the Christians wash away original sin through baptism. A person's soul is clean and regenerated after being dunked in the water. The ritual is held to give new life, to signal a rebirth. Going back even further in history, we find that the great deluge was the symbol of a great cleansing. It suggests great chaos and instantaneous dissolution through which Mother water takes back her children into herself and then produces rebirth.

Over the ages water has also been considered medically therapeutic. The Romans used their baths quite extensively, and many Native Americans felt the hot springs to be sacred places that could help cure physical ills.

Today the Europeans highly respect hydrotherapy, using warm or cold water to help cure colds, sore throats, fevers, arthritis, rheumatism, gout, nervousness, and many other diseases. Hydrotherapy remains a predominantly European method but holds less credibility in North America.

Although water in its various properties has been used for many centuries, only recently has it undergone scientific evaluation. These investigations were motivated primarily by the space flight programs, which researched the physiology of human immersion in water.

A paper in the *British Medical Journal* entitled "Observations on the Effects of Immersion in Bath Spa Water," reported that immersion in water (35° C) produced profound physiological changes, including increased cardiac output, excretion of urine, potassium, and sodium. The blood pressure, however, remained constant. These changes, showing that simple immersion in water can have beneficial effects on the body's processes, have become part of the scientific rationale for the spa treatment of many diseases.

Through its uses in relieving thirst, cooking, and cleaning, water satisfies the most basic needs in life. Yet it is a complex element, serving many diverse functions and constituting a symbol and a sacrament in religions throughout time. In this section we have glimpsed only a few of its special properties. In the next section, we will take a look at a characteristic that has emerged in the Western world only in the last three decades: its ability to facilitate labor and birth.

THE PHYSICAL AND CULTURAL ORIGINS OF WATER BIRTH

The physical development of an individual is said to reflect that of a whole species. The evolution of a human embryo also seems to recapitulate the development of life on earth.

At its earliest stage, the fertilized human ovum is a single-celled creature, much like the single cells of the first life forms on earth during the Cambrian period. As the embryo develops, it is virtually indistinguishable from that of a multicelled animal like a sponge; then it resembles a fish, then an amphibian, then a primitive mammal, and finally it takes a truly human form. Interestingly, at one point during fetal development the human fetus is very similar to the dolphin or whale fetus, sharing the same sort of tail and general physiognomy. Perhaps, given the way the fetus recapitulates evolutionary history, including the whole first period of evolution on the seas, the human baby at birth still carries some of the aquatic abilities of its progenitors.

Professor Sir Alister Hardy, a marine biologist, has posited an aquatic stage during human evolution (1960), based on the work of Professor Wood Jones, who wrote of the vestigial hairs that remain on the human body. The human fetus, especially in the premature child, has a covering of fine lanugo hair whose arrangement perfectly depicts the lines that the flow of water would follow over the human body. These patterns were adapted for the purposes of streamlining through the water, and eventually, through evolution, they were discarded. Hardy suggests that, unlike our cousin the chimpanzee, we have lost our hair because of our aquatic period, and, as the aquatic mammals do, we have taken on subcutaneous fat instead of hair in order to keep ourselves warm. Hardy, quoting Jones's book, cites the difference in the subcutaneous fat of the human species as compared to that of any other primate and reminds us of the layers of blubber on the whale, seals, and penguins, as well as other water animals. In warm-blooded water mammals this layer of fat prevents heat loss, replacing the function of the hair.

The human's erect posture is another factor to take into consideration. The chimpanzee slouches forward, supporting the weight of his torso with his long arms, whereas humans are able to stand erect. Perhaps slowly over the ages humans went deeper and deeper into the water and had to adopt an erect posture in order to keep their heads above the water. In order to eat, humans could stand on the bottom while the water kept them buoyant and afloat. Hardy argues that the sensitivity in our fingertips may be due to our ancestors' need to grope through cloudy waters for food such as fish and shellfish. After human balance improved, they learned to stand on shore and then eventually could run. Humans would return to shore to sleep and to get water.

Hardy hypothesizes that the "missing link" may perhaps be found in the oceans and seas. He asks, "Where are the fossil remains that linked the Hominidae with their more ape-like ancestors? The finds in South Africa of Australopithecus seem to carry us a good step nearer to our common origin with the ape stock, but before then there is a gap" (1960, p. 651). He suggests that humans died in the sea, leaving their remains to be ground up by powerful sea creatures or to be eroded away by the tropical seas. Hardy reminds us that at present a great gap exists in the geological record of early human history. This is a period of a million years for which no fossil remains of early humans have been found. Did our ancestors just disappear? Or do they remain at the bottom of the seas, yet to be discovered?

Elaine Morgan took Hardy's ideas even further in her books, *The Descent of Woman* (1972) and *The Aquatic Ape* (1982). She postulates that our ancient ancestors returned to the waters millions of years ago and remained there for a few million years. In her works Morgan takes us back to the pre-Pleistocene era, the era that ostensibly produced Homo sapiens. In the very early Pleistocene period, the hominids that were dug up in the Olduvai Gorge were already using tools and walking on their hind legs. This era was preceded by the hot, desertlike Pliocene, and before the Pliocene came the mild Miocene, which produced the Proconsul, a primate whose remains have been dug up in large numbers. The Miocene also produced a vegetarian prehominid hairy ape who lived in the trees, obtaining her food and sleeping while up there. She also spent part of her time on the ground.

In the Pliocene era, the climate changed drastically to desert conditions on the African continent that had extreme heat waves, bringing droughts and replacing trees with scrub and grass. Having no trees to escape to or to find food in, the prehominid ape was forced to live in the open savannah. Her limbs were accustomed not to walking but to gripping, thereby placing her at a disadvantage for escaping the carnivorous cats that found her to be easy prey now that she had left the trees. During most of her adult life, she was encumbered with babies, suckling, or being pregnant, which did not make for an easy escape since primate babies are slow developers. When a predator was after her, her only escape was the vast area of water where the predator would not go, especially since he could adapt even less than she to standing on his hind feet. She could go out farther than her predator without drowning since she could go up to her neck. While there, she discovered that it was pleasantly cooler in the water and she could find shellfish, crabs, and other little delicacies that the savannah could not provide.

The human was not the only land-dwelling creature that returned to the water. Seventy million years ago, the cetaceans (the porpoises, dolphins, and whales) were some of the first mammals to return to the sea. Then, 50 million years ago, relatives of the elephants took to the water; their descendants are the sea cows or the sirenians. A bearlike creature, a carnivore, took to the sea 25 to 30 million years ago and became the present-day walruses, fur seals, and sea lions. In *The Aquatic Ape,* Morgan stated: "Most surviving mammalian orders include species which took to the water, and then evolved specific adaptations for aquatic life. One of the few orders which is generally believed to include no such species is the Primates—to which man belongs" (p. 25).

The aquatic ape theory accounts for the extreme differences between Homo sapiens and all the other apes. Man did not lose hair because he was a perspiring hunter, but because it kept him cold in the water. Instead, he developed the layer of subcutaneous fat, which maintains greater warmth in the water than is possible with a layer of hair on the outside. Hair traps air and insulates in that fashion. On a full aquatic mammal, all the hair has been lost, for fur would be a handicap, slowing down the streamlined effect. Competitive swimmers sometimes shave their body hair in order to become more streamlined, which enables them to glide through the water faster.

Our only remaining hair is on top of our heads. According to the *National Geographic Magazine* of March 1975 the women of Tierra del

Fuego spend long periods of time in the water, and their children hang onto their mother's hair. Morgan points out that other aquatic mammals do not have long heads of hair, because their offspring are descendants of mammals with hoofs and claws. They had nothing to grasp with, even if there had been hair on top of the mother's heads. Even today, women find that their hair grows much thicker during pregnancy. This thickness is not intended to enhance sexual attraction; after all, after conception takes place, why would nature try to increase sexual attractiveness? Rather, this thick hair could be one of the remaining memories of our aquatic life when our children hung onto our hair when they grew tired while in the water.

Igor Charkowsky speaks of the breath-hold reflex that all humans are born with and soon lose owing to their lack of a continued water existence. Charkowsky starts swimming training minutes after the baby is born. He dunks the babies into the water and brings them up immediately. While under water, the newborns make the same motions that they did in the womb, as any mother watching can testify. These motions are swimming motions. When the newborns are free to float and glide through the water, they start kicking like little frogs while holding their breath.

Elaine Morgan observes that man possess some of the same physiological diving adaptations as those of the aquatic mammals. Trained breath-hold divers or pearl divers have been known to dive to 262 feet, while the harbor porpoise dives 66 feet, the penguin 150 feet, and the blue whale 330 feet. The duration of the dives is 3.5 minutes for man, 0.5 minute for the puffin, 10 minutes for the walrus, and 75 minutes for the sperm whale. The diving reflex, which humans have in common with aquatic mammals, includes a reduction in heart rate (bradycardia) and cardiac output, which results from the action of the vagus nerve and reduces the body's consumption of oxygen. While diving, the penguin has a heartbeat of 20 beats per minute (BPM); before diving, the penguin has 200 BPM. The human's BPM upon diving is 35 and before diving, 72 BPM. A sea lion's BPM is 20 upon diving and 95 before diving, while the Beluga is 12 to 20 BPM during and 100 before the dive.

Morgan reports a conversation with a swimming instructor in Los Angeles who felt that swimming comes naturally to babies at a very early age and if, after ten months, the babies have not swum, they forget what was once a natural motion and action for them. Morgan points out that, in their first year of life, babies like to be in the water and are not afraid to stick their heads under the water. I myself have trained many babies to swim, and I have observed the same situation: the sooner they are introduced to the water, the more they like it and the more willing they are to accept it. The later they are introduced to the water, the more difficult it is for them to adapt to the water. I have also found this to be true even in babies who were taught to swim shortly after birth, but whose lessons were not kept up: after the first year, these toddlers will have a difficult time even putting their faces in the water.

In *The Aquatic Ape* (1982), Morgan also quotes the organizer for the Edinburgh County Council at the Royal Commonwealth Pool who states that during their first year of life children have an inborn reflex that stops them from breathing for short periods of time while under the water. During these times no water gets into the lungs. After the first year, however, they lose this breath-hold reflex.

Before leaving Elaine Morgan, let us discuss one last point she makes: there are differences in mammalian copulation. Morgan notes that most terrestrial mammals approach and copulate from behind, whereas the aquatic mammals copulate belly to belly, much as the hairless terrestrial mammals known as humans. As an example, Morgan cites the extinct Steller's Sea Cow. This species has been seen playfully rolling about in the water with other of its kind and playing many love games. The male deceives the female by making many twists and turns, an activity that bores the female. Eventually, she tires of his games and lies on her back in the water, which brings the male rushing to her, embracing in the ventro-ventral position. Morgan points out that all the aquatic mammals that copulate in the ventro-ventral position have terrestrial ancestors.

Dolphins and whales have become a subject of great interest and study as a result of the attention which the mass slaughtering of these intelligent creatures produced. Anyone who has gazed on the waters of the northern Pacific Ocean from November until February can see the gray whale making one of the longest migrations recorded of any mammal. It is an inspiring sight. A week after the first water birth that I attended, I drove down to the middle of the Baja Peninsula in Mexico to whale watch. Going from the water birth of a land mammal to that of an aquatic mammal seemed to form a wonderful continuum for me. I arrived at Scammon's Lagoon, where I saw the huge creatures dancing with a grace that even Baryshnikov could not match. I sat on the beach transfixed while the great beings hurtled themselves into the air as if they were hot air balloons rising to the sky. Some would spin themselves in the air like a top, and others stood on their heads in the water minutes at a time, with their great tail fins sticking out of the water like monuments commemorating their great journey from the north. They reminded me of children walking on their hands on the bottom of a swimming pool with their feet wiggling in the air. The grays' happiness and playfulness soon became catching, and I found myself attempting to do cartwheels on the beach to join in the fun.

From there, I traveled to the sleepy little coastal town of Guerrero

Negro, where the whales came so close to the docks that I could look these beautiful creatures right in the eye. The eyes of these giants reflected nothing but gentleness, peacefulness, and a very ancient wisdom. One mother floated by with her newborn calf close enough for me to see the milk squirting out in the water. The milk looked rich and creamy as the little one fed while gliding by. I could not imagine how anyone could kill these gentle souls. Now that my water birth experience had reached full circle, I left Baja to research human and cetacean water births.

I found the comparison that Elaine Morgan made about the copulation of humans and aquatic mammals worth researching; while during this work, I also came across literature on the parturition of dolphins and whales. Many resources wrote about the playfulness and the prolonged love play that precedes these animals' final act of copulation. Both the male and female display many acts of great tenderness, and the female plays a very active role. Since the male cannot smell the female in estrus, she shows it through play and affection, signaling the male that it is time to make babies.

Many women clients and friends have confided to me that during the time of ovulation, they become so aroused that they cannot keep their hands off their lovers. While none of the fathers that I have worked with reported that they could "smell" when their wives were ovulating, as one father put it, "She sure gets a lot friendlier!"

Even more fascinating are the births of the dolphins and whales who are attended in labor by their own "midwives." The newborns must be able to swim immediately after birth and to maintain their body temperature. They are not able to go to a cave or a nest for safekeeping or warmth. The newborn cetacean must have fairly large dimensions, weighing in at birth at 5 to 6 percent of the mother's weight in rorquals and 10 to 15 percent in dolphins. There is a correlation between the length of gestation and the size of the young at birth, with the average time of gestation for most Cetacea being between ten and twelve months and for sperm and pilot whales sixteen months. They occasionally have twins. The prenatal mortality of the fetus is higher with older mothers; the fetuses are reabsorbed into the mother's system when they die.

All cetaceans are born with a tail presentation, which is unusual for most uniparous mammals (giving birth to one offspring at a time) whose head usually presents first. Parturition for the Cetacea lasts from twenty-five minutes to two hours. The birth of a bottlenose dolphin has been reported to take five minutes. As long as the placenta supplies sufficient oxygen, there is no danger that the young will be forced to breathe—except if the umbilical cord is stretched tight, is in a knot, is pressed, or the blood flow is impeded in some other way. Since the fetus

is born tail first, the blowhole is last to emerge, and even in a complicated delivery the calf is not likely to inhale too much water. (*Author's
note:* Charkowsky believes that breech births in human babies are safer
in the water since the bottom half of the fetus is not cold; therefore, the
newborn is not gasping in amniotic fluid while the head is still inside
the mother.)

In baleen whales the umbilical cord is about 40 percent as long as
the newborn and in toothed whales it is about 45 to 50 percent. The
length tells us that it is immaterial whether the cetacean is born head
or tail first, since the cord is long enough for either end to come out
first. The cord is long enough, so that the blowhole can be at the surface
when the baby takes its first breath. The newborn faces the danger of
inspiring fluid, if it does not go to the surface.

A report by Lockley (1979) of a bottlenose dolphin during the last few
days of pregnancy told of being able to detect fetal movements. The
number of the mother's defecations increased as the day of birth approached, as did her respirations. During the last few days, the mother
stayed near the surface of the water because when labor begins, the
mothers cannot swim very fast.

The description of the exit of the fetus is as remarkable as that of a
human's. In the birth process, the fins and the flippers fold in perfectly
and fit into the mother's depressions, so that they easily slide out. When
the newborn is completely out, the umbilical cord breaks as the baby
swims to the surface; if it fails to break, the mother pushes it to the
surface. The placenta is expelled 0.5 to 10 hours after the birth. It is
never eaten, and it sinks to the bottom. Morgan points out that humans
also do not eat their placentas.

The calves are lovingly cared for not only by their mothers, but also
by the other cetaceans. At the time of birth, another female is always
present, acting as a midwife. If the mother does not get the calf to the
surface on time, the midwife will help. The midwife will also help get
out a dead calf by tugging at it, or it will get the placenta out by tugging
at the umbilical cord.

Being true mammals, cetaceans nurse their young. The mammary
glands are situated in slits on each side of the genital opening and
protrude slightly when the mother is lactating. The calves are always
suckled under water, though close to the surface. The mother is said to
move very slowly and then to roll to the side so that the young may
grab hold of the nipple with the tongue and the tip of the palate. They
are not equipped to suck. Whale milk is three to four times the concentration of the terrestrial mammal's milk. The content is 40 to 50 percent
fat and 11 to 12 percent protein. The fat content of land mammals
ranges from 2 to 17 percent.

Breastfeeding lasts from four to fourteen months, depending on the species. The maternal love and care lasts much longer, possibly for life in some species. If a calf is orphaned at an early age, other members of the pod will take over its care.

In daily life, the young are closely cared for and will be aggressively defended by the whole pod if in danger. Gray whales have been called "devilish" for their aggressive defenses. The calves even have "babysitters" while the mother goes out in search of food. It is a joy to watch the young hitching rides on the bow waves or convection currents that the adults make. The young hardly have to move their flukes to keep up with the group.

Most of the literature depicts the cetaceans as a very caring, community-based group. We resemble our giant cousins in many ways and could perhaps learn more about our past, be it aquatic or 100 percent terrestrial, through further study of this wise mammalian race.

Interested in discovering any other cultures, past or present, that used water for laboring or delivering, I searched through the Human Relations Area Files (HRAF) that were organized according to country or tribe.[1] There I found corroboration of information from my former midwife partner, Claudia Ford, who on a visit of the Panamanian Islands discussed water births with the Cuna women. Cuna women have a most interesting approach to water births: "Shortly before the baby is to be born, a hole is cut in the hammock through which the baby passes and drops into a Cayuca filled with sea water or a medicine bath. The work of the medicine man is then over and it is up to the midwife to care for both mother and child in such a way that both may enjoy good health."[2] Another account states:

> Birth takes place in the house within an improvised enclosure from which children and men are excluded. An innatuledi, who remains outside the enclosure, chants and supplies the childbirth medicines according to the report of progress given from time to time by the midwife who is inside with the mother. The child is born into a water-filled canoe which is placed beneath the hammock in which the mother lies. The midwife removes the umbilical cord and buries it in the floor of the house. Both husband and wife observe several taboos during pregnancy and the husband observes a mild couvade in that he keeps to the house for three days after the birth.
>
> While the midwives pass to and fro from partition to shaman, the girl's parents stolidly wait; the young husband paces back and forth. Labor is frequently prolonged and may bring unconsciousness. Shortly before birth a hole is cut in the woman's hammock; through this the baby drops to a canoe filled with sea water or medicine placed below. Sterilization is an unknown concept, and when the baby splashes into the cool water, the midwives rescue it and swaddle it with old cloths. This ends the shamans'

responsibility; now the midwives must care for the mother and new child. A midwife buries the afterbirth in the floor of the house.

The hours dragged by like years until the fateful hour of midnight was at hand; fearful and with bated breath the family waited. The old grandmother rocked back and forth in her corner; the father and mother stoically stared into space; and the young husband walked aimlessly up and down, mutely weeping and wringing his hands. Hark! What sound was that which broke the pulsing silence? Was there a splash? Yes, for a feeble wail filled the little hut.

A new life had entered this earthly sphere by way of emersion, for true to Indian custom, Sepu's baby was allowed to fall into a canoe of water which had been prepared beneath her hammock. In contrast to the warm olive oil bath which modern science gives to more fortunate little babes, she was treated to a breath-taking plunge into cold water. Quickly, she was rescued by one of the midwives and wrapped in old rags, for the San Blas mother-to-be prepares no layette previous to birth. Then she was carried out to the eager family where she was almost smothered with attention. How quickly the scene in the outer room had changed from one of deepest gloom to almost uncontrollable joy! Sepu's grandmother showed her shrunken gums in a toothless grin of ecstasy, her parents fondled the baby, and the pride enveloped young father sat near a flickering light and immediately began to work on a tiny dress for his firstborn in order to quiet his nerves![3]

These selections about the Cuna were reported by male anthropologists, who because of the taboos of Cuna society were unable to personally observe the labor and delivery of the Cuna woman. They had to rely on informants who also may have been men and may not have gotten the true picture.

While researching childbirth in different cultures, I came upon a book titled *Human Birth: An Evolutionary Perspective* by Wenda R. Trevathan (1987). As Trevathan was searching through HRAF and through other reports that contained information on childbirth, she found that, out of 296 reports, in only 22 sources (nineteen cultures) had the writers of the reports actually witnessed the delivery. Apparently, many cultures uphold the modesty of birth. In many cultures it is taboo for a stranger, especially men, to be present at a birth. Most anthropologists have had to rely on informants, thereby making the information inadequate or inaccurate. In the Philippines one male anthropologist was killed when he was caught secretly trying to observe a birth. One anthropologist wrote of the difficulty of obtaining information about birth since the subject is restricted to women. Even Margaret Mead had trouble when she first went to Manus in 1928. She found that only women who had given birth could be present at a birth, and so Mead had to rely on information from informants. Mead observed that in fieldwork it is important not to deceive one's informants, especially when the truth is sought. Her account of that study was unremarkable as regards childbirth. However, in 1956, when she returned to Manus after she herself had given birth, she was able to observe and study birthing at close range. Her study notes many details of the activities of the mother, midwives, and those present at the birth.

Trevathan also states that just because a person is witness to a birth the account is not necessarily accurate. Until recently, few anthropologists (who were mostly men) were interested only in what was done with the placenta and how the umbilical cord was cut. Only recently, with the influx of women interested in reporting the minutiae of the birthing process, have vast improvements occurred in the information gathered. This author took a midwifery course in El Paso, Texas, so that she would have a better understanding of what she was observing.

While attending the first Under Water Birth Conference in Tutukaka, New Zealand in 1982, I met a Maori woman, Cammy, who described how the ancestral Maori women would give birth in the warm waters of Rotorua where there are naturally occurring hot springs. The Maoris have considered the area and the springs to be sacred. Cammy gave birth in a large European-size bathtub and experienced a beautiful water birth. When I looked in the Maori section in HRAF, I basically found information on umbilical cord cuttings and only a few statements on childbirth. There were no data whatever on water birth. The documents that were in the files were old and contained sketchy information with few details. Whatever the reason for the paucity of information on laboring or water births, we cannot exclude water birth as a viable means for a woman having a wonderful nonmedicated labor and delivery.

In a conversation with Michel Odent at his home in London, I learned of a water birth that took place in a village in France in 1805 as reported in the *Annales dela Société de Médecine Pratique de Montpellier*. Eager to read the article myself, I wrote to Jacques Gelis, a historian with access to the article in Etampes, France. The article was in French, and, alas, being the typical American that I am, I am illiterate in French. A friend, Margaret Ewing, who has spoken French fluently for more than thirty years, kindly translated the work for me.

A WATER BIRTH IN 1805

Do obstetricians today who recommend a convivial birth in the swimming pool know that about two centuries ago some of their colleagues had already tried the virtue of water?

When he was called to the bedside of Mme. de L. in early 1805, Dr. Embry, an associate of the Society of Practical Medicine of Montpellier, practicing at Aubenas, was far from realizing that his services would make him a precursor. The "gentlewoman," 28 or 30 years old, had had a "good pregnancy." Nothing indicated the difficulties of a birth she considered as coming late.

The morning after the first pains, she was surrounded by "people who had promised to look after her." The "twinges," the first pains heralding labor, only increased. Visits from her friends doubled her calm reassurance. She was prescribed douches and was made to take violet water and a little broth now and then.

At the end of the day, heavy pains came on; the lady noticed the difference; her calm was increased by new sensations of which she had been warned, and delivery seemed imminent. The pains doubled, and the doctor asked the midwife to examine the patient to estimate the state of her labor. The midwife said that she was well dilated, and she predicted a natural birth. In this comfortable environment in a small town in Haut Lanquedoc, it was the usual practice to call in the midwife; but the doctor remained in charge, ready to intervene in case of any complications.

Between pains, the woman, supported by her helpers, walked a little around the room, sat in an armchair or on the edge of the bed, and seemed quite "normal." However, toward 11:00 at night, her pains weakened, and being tired, she fell asleep. She slept for two hours when she was awakened by strong pains. Her attendants thought she was about to deliver. The doctor examined her carefully; the matrix seemed "soft to him and very small." He added, "I seemed to perceive parts of the child's lower limbs, and I began to suspect the birth might not take place unaided. Judging by the length of labor, I attempted to find by touch its progression. I found the orifice completely dilated without tension or pain; the dimensions quite adequate, the position of the head quite natural; my finger could trace part of its circumference, the head came up with a slight effort. The pains, apparently stronger, however gave it no progress."

The obstetrician wondered, but he said nothing. On the contrary, he urged the woman to have patience and, above all, not to push uselessly. Then he made an excuse to leave them for a moment. He went to a friend's house to beg him to send urgently for the obstetrician of Vallon Pont d'Arc, a town more than 30 kilometers away; but the roads were bad and at best he could not count on help for twelve hours. The doctor then returned to the woman in labor and took advantage of the conversation to explain the action he felt might be necessary.

A day had gone by now, and the labor still had not progressed. He ordered a douche and, in the evening, bleeding. The woman seemed better for it and continued to be brave and calm. A surgeon was called and after examining her confirmed the inertia of the matrix and noted that red phlegm flowed now and then. At the end of the day some vapor appeared; the doctor gave her a spoonful of an antispasmodic potion that brought back the heavy pains, "the last of which seemed strong enough to end labor."

In the evening, the messenger sent to Vallon came back. The obstetrician was sick and could not travel. The doctor was greatly disappointed.

"It was difficult for me to keep up the conversational tone," he affirmed, "however, it was indispensable to establish my assurance of the end of the labor." The doctor now called in a colleague who was too old to practice, but nonetheless was a careful man with good judgment. He told his colleague of his plan, and the old doctor agreed. The doctor knew he could not count on surgery in this particular case, because, although he owned a forceps, he had never been taught how to use it. He did not dare to use it himself, "not having followed that course" when he left the Boudelcogne school some years before, "although," he added, "this seemed to me the best instrument to turn the child to make the delivery by the feet." The doctor instead relied on the aid of the local doctor in the small town. "The small town doctors, with their own ideas, deprived of the help their colleagues can give them in surgery, pharmacy, and medicine, who have never dared attempt grave medical operations can well understand my perplexity."

Labor was weakening, and the woman had to be helped to end a situation that was becoming more difficult every hour. "False pains" tormented her cruelly, and soon despair overcame this woman who had been so calm and courageous until now. Her mother, too, had been unable to deliver without help, and she now feared she would be unable to deliver herself. "She was lost, her face fell in and her features showed despair and distress."

In a firm voice, the doctor announced his intention to "trying a bath." That is, to have the woman deliver in water. He added that they still had all medical resources if necessary, in case water proved useless. He did not say what gave him the idea of the bath, nor did he talk at any time of rupturing the membranes. But he had noticed, by touch, the dryness and soreness of the vagina and thus wished to moisten those parts to aid the exit of the child. Thus orders to prepare the bath were given and Madame finally decided to be put in it despite the prejudices and unwillingness of the helpers. Soon the false pains died down, "her expression revived and there followed a quarter of an hour of calm. I felt the lower abdomen meanwhile," continued the doctor, "and the matrix seemed to me to get back its firmness." This was the first gleam of hope after two days of anxiety. All at once, Madame sat up and wanted to leave the bath. A true pain had came on, and it terrified her. After being prevented from leaving the bath, she agreed that this pain was more supportable and she pushed harder. I then announced that she would deliver in the bath. The pains continued and her courage revived. Each pain increased with effects not produced by those before it. Finally something was happening. I asked the surgeon on my right to feel her. The head had crossed the passage! Madame was calm and waited quietly for the pains to expel the trunk. They came quickly. The baby announced itself with hearty cries as soon as it left the water. The afterbirth was soon expelled by new contractions. I helped them with gentle massage and Madame was straight way taken from the bath.

Forty-eight hours had passed during labor, and the doctor ended his report: "The effects of this birth were not remarkable. Madame and her son, at this time, are in the best of health."[4]

THE RUSSIAN INFLUENCE

In the twentieth century, the Russians have been the innovators of quite a few methods of childbirth. The Lamaze method originated in Russia, which originally was termed *psychoprophylaxis*. Dr. Fernand Lamaze brought it to France and popularized it throughout many parts of the Western world.

Another method that has come to us from Russia is the water birth method. Igor Charkowsky pioneered the method in the early 1960s after his daughter was born prematurely at seven months gestation. Apparently, she weighed only 1.2 kilograms at birth (2.64 pounds). Even with today's technology, this baby would be considered a miracle baby. While the doctors gave her up for hopeless, Charkowsky placed her in what he called a water environment, returning her to a world where she was safe. Charkowsky claims that his daughter spent most of the first two years of her life in a water environment. Today the child is a happy, healthy, and intelligent woman.

As noted earlier, I first met Charkowsky in Moscow in 1986. My only contact who was to take me to Charkowsky was someone I had never met before, and all I knew about him was a telephone number. At that time, the then Soviet Union required that all foreign visitors check into an Intourist Hotel. To receive a telephone call from an outsider was chancy, and the conversation had to be kept to polite conversation, for Charkowsky, I soon discovered, was being watched. When I arrived in the Moscow airport, I went directly to my hotel and tried phoning my contact. There was no answer. I tried again later and still no answer. It was a beautiful full moon night, and Red Square was not far from my hotel. So why not take a walk? Upon leaving my room, I noticed a woman sitting at the end of the hall at a desk and walked past her. In a heavily accented English, she yelled at me to stop. As I approached her, she glared at me and asked me where I was going. My American sense of freedom got a bit ruffled, and I politely inquired why she needed to know. She reminded me of the women in the 1940s detective movies that I had watched when I was a kid—tough and hard boiled. She explained to me that I must sign out and I must sign in, and where was I going anyway? A foreigner was not to go to places that were not sanctioned, she reminded me, and I could only be accompanied by an official if I was going somewhere without my tour. "What tour?" I thought. I then told her I was only going down to the lobby, but when I got there I slipped out the front door of the hotel without any problems. I surmised that they had many rules, but they simply didn't have enough people to enforce them.

It was a hot summer's night. A clock pointed to midnight. The streets were filled with people singing, some of them dancing and others just sitting in the park and talking. It was as if it was twelve noon instead of midnight. I looked up at the beautiful full moon as I headed to Red Square. As I approached the Kremlin, the moon and the Red Star over the Kremlin were perfectly aligned. It was a beautiful sight until I thought about what the Red Star symbolized.

The square was an architectural beauty with its red cobblestones and the gay-colored domes of St. Basil's Cathedral at the far end. Since I was so obviously a Westerner, many people came up to me trying to use their English. Fortunately most spoke English very well, which was great as I spoke no Russian.

The next morning the phone rang: it was my contact making arrangements to take me to Charkowsky. He told me to meet him at the stairs leading to the front door of the hotel in one hour. When we met, he hailed a taxi, and off we went to meet Charkowsky at one of the embassies.

On arriving at the embassy, a door flew open, and Charkowsky greeted me with open arms and a warm embrace. His lecture was just about to begin, and I was seated near the front, giving me the opportunity to glance around the room. Everyone was dressed in suits and ties and seemed to come from all walks of life. The lecture was in Russian. Charkowsky speaks no English and only a bit of German. An interpreter was therefore provided for me. Charkowsky seemed just as interested in getting information about childbirth from me as I was from him.

I was with Charkowsky until the wee hours of the morning. With him were many people interested in his work: pediatricians, nuclear physicists, artists, journalists, physiologists, midwives, doctors from almost every branch of medicine, and even a Tibetan monk. Charkowsky collaborates with some of Moscow's leading psychics (or as the Russians call them, "sensitives") at births, and when working as a healer.

I often wondered if Charkowsky ever slept, for while I was with him, we were in constant motion. Once we went to the large natatorium, where babies not yet able to crawl were swimming like fish, seemingly more at home in the water than on land. The older children, ages 2 to 4, were jumping off the edge of the pool, diving to the bottom, then getting out, and quickly doing it all over again. These children seemed very capable and happy. They also appeared to be strong and well adapted to spending a lot of time in the water.

Sometimes we would jump on the metro, Moscow's underground train system, where the walls were made of beautiful marble, with no trace of graffiti on them. Commemorative statues were all over Moscow, and the underground was no exception. The crystal chandeliers that had once belonged in a palace were now on the underground, clean and untouched.

Charkowsky makes use of his now famous plexiglass tank for people to birth in and to teach their newborns to swim. The tank was transported all over Moscow and was either waiting for a woman to go into labor or was being used for teaching babies to swim. Always we were warmly greeted with food and chi (tea) generously shared. A beautiful table was always set, even though these people had so little by American standards.

The babies were dunked up and down in the water and let go for a few seconds. They would kick their little feet like frogs, and the stronger ones would lift their heads up for air. Most of the time the mothers brought the babies quickly to the surface. In these homes, around the brightly adorned dinner tables, we would exchange information until the early hours of the morning. I taped all the conversations, and here I would like to present summaries of a small portion of the talks that took place in Moscow and the Black Sea area in 1987.

Charkowsky believes that "Childbirth is a very intimate thing. During childbirth, only mother and father should be present."[5] Charkowsky opposes anyone else being there, except the midwives. He does only homebirths and there is no clinic. He said that the Swedish documentary about him misrepresented him in that respect. Either he or the families take the tank around to the homes where the next water birth will happen.

Charkowsky claims to be a sensitive/healer. He also claims to be able to move energies. While I was working with him, I was astonished to witness his ability to turn a breech baby to the head-down position—without touching the mother. He waved his hands above the mother as if he were massaging her belly from the air. The belly started rippling, and after a time the baby was in the head-down position. I felt the position before and after, and there was definitely a difference. Perhaps this was a coincidence, perhaps not.

Charkowsky grew up in a village near the Russian-Chinese border. His grandmother was a sensitive, and his parents were shamans who practiced folk medicine. Apparently, a long line of his ancestors practiced folk medicine. Russia is rich with folk medicine from village to village. Some traditions indeed appear to be superstitions, whereas others are folk remedies that have been handed down from generation to generation. Owing to the expansiveness of the country and the remoteness of many villages, this way of life has been maintained into modern times. As a child, Charkowsky played with the dolphins at the seaside, which led to his lifelong involvement with these gentle creatures. He believes that dolphins can speak to us psychically.

Charkowsky said that he had visions of Ancient Egypt, where the high priestesses helped birth the royalty in the water. He also told a story about his grandmother's work with premature infants. At one time she saved a 7-month-old fetus by putting him in a sheep's bladder sac filled with milk. The baby survived and was healthy, although the doctors had given him up for dead. Charkowsky explains: "It is wrong to put a child in a position where there is gravitational pull on immature tissue and immature blood system and circulatory system." "This," he says, "is against the normal physiology. If the child is put in water the gravitational pull will not affect him. The baby should be given conditions as to where he formerly was—the water."[6]

Charkowsky claimed to have attended over one thousand water births as of 1986. His work has now expanded to many parts of the former USSR including St. Petersburg and the Crimea. Working with babies being born in the water is not as phenomenal for him as it is to most other people. His main interest is teaching babies to swim. Every year he journeys to the Black Sea on the Crimean Peninsula near the famous resort town of Yalta. Charkowsky asked Nathaniel and me if we would like to join them the next summer (1987) in birthing babies in the sea and also teaching babies to swim.

By the time the summer of 1987 rolled around, Nathaniel had turned 3 and we were on our way to Yalta, a beautiful town with nice beaches and a boardwalk that probably looks much the same today as in 1945 when the Big Three divided up the world between them. Charkowsky and a few of our other friends from Moscow, as well as a member of the World Health Organization, met us when we arrived in Yalta. Charkowsky was there to observe the births of the babies and to participate in teaching the babies to swim.

After a few days, we left Yalta to journey to the camp near Sudak, where others were awaiting our arrival. At the camp, far from any sandy beach, we found only a rocky shore and a place with no facilities. We cooked our food over fires and slept in tents that were cushioned by seaweed that had dried from lying on the beach. Little children could be seen bobbing up and down in the Black Sea, looking ever so much like little sea nymphs. Pregnant mothers walked around in their bikinis, showing their beautiful big bellies. Charkowsky's two sons were playing in the water; they were much older since their depiction in the *Water Babies* book (1982). Nathaniel immediately began to play with the other children; the language difference was no barrier at their age. They spoke to each other in their own tongues and seemed to understand each other completely.

While at the Black Sea, the families swam daily. The pregnant mothers, swimming alongside real dolphins only a few meters away, copied the movements of the dolphins. At times no distinction could be made between human and dolphin.

A few of the midwives with whom Charkowsky had worked were swimming with their children. Some of the children were barely able to walk, but they took to the water like ducks. Tanya and Sveta, though not sanctioned by the Ministry of Health, were some of the traditional midwives. I might add, they were two of the most knowledgeable and competent midwives I have met anywhere in the world.

The days were filled with information exchanges that continued long into the night. Charkowsky spoke of a scientist named Constantine Salkowsky

> whose dreams were of living in space, of the future of cosmonauts. When Salkowsky's work was discovered by the authorities, they burned it because there was mention of mystics in his writings. Salkowsky's work was written about 100 years ago. His ideas were to be living in space for the future people. He believed that humankind should go into cosmic areas. When I became familiar with these ideas, I understood that people should be going through the water milieu because the water medium is a step toward zero gravity.[7]

From what I could understand, this seemed to be one of the basic premises on which Charkowsky founded his belief in water birth and infant swimming. I sometimes wondered what was being lost in the translation, although his translators were very fluent in English and also worked with him closely. They understood his work almost as well as he did. While working with Charkowsky, I tried to make no prejudgments. I felt that I was there much as an anthropologist would be there—to observe, take notes, record, and learn.

Charkowsky postulates that the brain of a baby is one-seventh of its body weight. In contrast the brain of an adult is only 2 percent of total body weight. This suggests that, under the conditions of gravity, more energy is required for the baby to live and priority is given to the development of such elements as lungs, stomach, and the digestion and secretion organs. A larger brain requires a more powerful energy supply system. Charkowsky reminds us that we have evolved in a liquid environment in the womb. In a traditional gravitational setting, the fetus must fight to adapt itself to push a relatively large and extremely vulnerable brain through a comparatively narrow *sortie* (French for a fairly narrow going out) to withstand a tremendous gravitational blast and to inhale a giant's portion of the strongest oxidizer known as oxygen. Charkowsky likens an "air" birth to someone freefalling and then colliding with the solid ground. He tries to put the adult in the newborn's place by reminding us of the newborn's sensitivity. At such a crucial time, the newborn is abruptly alienated from the mother. Breathing is autonomous and unregulated, with the newborn thrown into this autonomy before the physiological adaptations of the body are ready to occur. In addition, compared to that of the womb, the environment is harsh, with bright lights, gross temperature, and humidity variables prevailing. These factors, Charkowsky feels, can put the newborn into a state that is close to deep stress. Within these first moments of life, sensitive brain cells collapse under the conditions of the high content of oxygen and strong irritants. The conditions of gravity ensure that only the toughest and crudest elements of the brain survive, while the most valuable and delicate ones collapse during the first minutes of life.

Leboyer has called our attention to the newborn's delicateness and sensitivity, and reminds us that we need to treat the newborns as just that—sensitive and delicate creatures. Charkowsky takes us a step further, telling us that the biological field and the psychic field of the newborn are just as delicate and sensitive, open, and extremely responsive to many different kinds of suggestions. He believes that water can be a buffer for the newborn's delicate and open energy fields. He assures us not to fear: the baby delivered under water will avoid the ill effects of the gravitational environment and preserve many of the brain cells that otherwise would be destroyed. The water milieu helps to create a healthy well-adjusted individual.

An associate of Charkowsky, Igor Smirnov, worked with Charkowsky for five years researching the psychosomatic development of the water babies. I met Dr. Smirnov in Moscow in 1986, when he had just received his Ph.D. in psychology from the University of Leningrad, now St. Petersburg. Smirnov told me that his observations of water babies showed him that

> their psychosomatic development is considerably ahead of the standard integral characteristics. He has observed some water babies begin to stand up and move around the age of 2–3 months, they understand the meaning of speech symbols and begin to speak much earlier than their coevals, they don't exhibit aggressiveness in their behavior, and they also display telepathic and other extrasensory abilities.[8]

Smirnov shared Charkowsky's opinions on gravity. The unadapted newborn's sudden exposure to the force of gravity is harmful for the child. He writes:

> The main advantage is that the psychological trauma which the child may develop during birth as a result of hypoxia and asphyxia can be abolished.

The first few minutes and hours of life of the newborn infant are of tremendous importance for its subsequent mental development, and the psychological homeostasis of the child which is formed during these first
moments of life is a unique matrix for subsequent development of mental
functions. Childbirth in water enables a smooth and stress-free transition
to be made from the liquid environment (amniotic fluid) into another liquid environment.[9]

Smirnov also states:

Dr. Jampolsky from Leningrad University showed in her scientific research that the psychological homeostasis of the child, formed during
these first moments of life, is a unique matrix for subsequent development of mental functions. . . . Dr. Jampolsky recorded the first cry of new
born babies (delivered in the usual way) and made a sonogram; then she
compared it with the sonograms of different physical sounds in nature
and found out that the first cry of a baby matches to the cry of adult
person when this person is very angry. This fact shows that the birth
experience gives negative impulse to the psychological homeostasis of a
child. During childbirth in the water the baby does not cry, but smiles;
that indicates its harmonious relations with the world which it has entered, and as a result of this, such a child has strong positive psychic
abilities and has no aggressive tendencies.[10]

According to Charkowsky, water births, followed by water training,
have certain benefits:

"The elimination of the gravitational pressure will aid to the opening of
the consciousness. Babies will be free of aggression, will be much more
altruistic and spiritual. They will remember their last incarnations and
there will be a breakthrough in human evolution that will help solve the
problems of the people in a most profound way."[11] . . . There are two layers of understanding. They are not so split, it is more difficult to distinguish between physiology and psychology in the infant as well as we do
in the adult. We can see very well how the smallest changes in physiology
are reflected in the psychology of the infant.[12]

Charkowsky spoke of pregnant women going under water for a minute or so at a time, an activity he refers to as "diving." Charkowsky
hypothesized that if

animals dive during the pregnancy, they trained their unborn children
to hypoxia, and their children were more talented in their ability to hold
their breath. Most problems concerning human birth arise because the
fetus is not trained to hypoxia, and when the labor is long, then the brains
are forced to a great degree, so a lot of brain cells are damaged. If the

labor becomes difficult and hard, the baby could become hypoxic during labor; if the mother had been doing her diving, then the baby would have less of a chance of trauma and less chance of internal hemorrhage to the brain.[13]

One day while I was working along the shore of the Black Sea, a pod of dolphins swam by. The sight of them sailing through the air as if they had wings held me spellbound, giving me the feeling that I was actually swimming in the sea with them. When I laughingly told Charkowsky about my blip out of reality and into the sea with the dolphins, he smiled and gave me the thumbs-up signal, meaning that was good. Questioning him further, he told me of the importance of meditating on dolphins—of being in psychic contact with them when pregnant and the importance for the babies. He claims that it is more important to be in psychic than in physical contact with the dolphins. "The unborn child," he claims, "is practically mediating all the time. This state of consciousness is in a very high spiritual area. The dolphin's level of consciousness is very close to the level of the unborn child."[14] Charkowsky believes that through the pregnant mother's meditative thoughts on dolphins, the fetus is in psychic contact with them. "Water babies that have contact with dolphins are very kind and altruistic. They don't have an element of revenge even when there has been some element of problem for the babies."[15]

> They [the dolphins] are telepathic. The dolphins educate the fetus through this telepathy. If you put the baby in China, it will adopt the Chinese language. So when the baby comes in contact with dolphins, it will have the dolphin tongue. The dolphins very strongly invite the baby and the parents to the sea. They have contact there [Natasha, Igor's wife, claims] that they contact as equals and so they want to contact. It is like falling in love—the dolphins with the baby. The dolphins are more clever in this respect than we.[16]

John Sutphen, a physician interested in the biological capabilities of cetaceans (dolphins and whales), writes of *echolocation,* as the dolphins' form of communication. This communication is three dimensional. The echo does not just come from the outer layer of the animal communicated to but permeates into the inner tissues and bones. The soft organs and surfaces within the animal receive the same degree of echo as the outer skin. The dolphin has to be constantly aware of the inner workings of other dolphins in order to recognize them and communicate. It stands to reason that a dolphin would be able to communicate on some level with the unborn baby. If Charkowsky's theory is correct, then the fetus would be able to receive the dolphin's communication and possibly benefit from learning from the dolphin.

While at the Black Sea, Charkowsky, the head of the maternal and infant division from the World Health Organization, and I organized an international group called WATER—the World Aquaculture for Therapy, Ecology, and Research. This organization is dedicated to researching, obtaining, and giving out information throughout the world. (We welcome any information or inquiries on water birth; please write to WATER, P.O. Box 26, Glen Ellen, Calif. 95442 U.S.A.)

These are the transliterations that I made from the many tapes I recorded on the beaches of the Crimea. Some of this material does not form as continuous a narrative as I would like. Still, because this is the crux of Charkowsky's theories on water birthing and infant swimming, it is important to share it with my readers, giving us all much food for thought. Much is owed to this man, whose trail-blazing findings have helped thousands of women to labor in water successfully and to give birth to their babies in as gentle a manner as possible.

THE FRENCH INFLUENCE

Another champion and pioneer of labor in water is Michel Odent, a French surgeon whom I met in the early 1980s while he was doing lecture tours on pregnancy and labor. In 1988, while doing research and lecturing in Europe, I visited Dr. Odent in London, where he now has a homebirth practice. When I arrived at his home, his first action was to show me the exact spot in his home where his son, Pascal, was born. We spent a lovely afternoon together taking Pascal for a stroll in the park, talking about birth and mutual friends. Michel Odent is a very likable, gentle man. Some women do not want men attending at their births, but if I had another baby, I would want him to be there. His manner is gentle and unobtrusive, yet one can sense his strong capabilities. He sees birth as a natural everyday process, not as some disease that a doctor can cure. Nor does he fear birth.

After our walk through the park, Dr. Odent took me to the flat where, during the day before, he had helped a couple give birth. They were the loveliest family, and Odent beamed with pride as he showed me the couple's new baby. He was so excited that one would have thought this was the first time he had been an attendant to a birth. On the way back to his flat, we chatted about how much more work it takes to attend homebirths than hospital or clinic births. I laughed and said, "Why Dr. Odent, you are becoming a midwife!" He looked at me as if I had just bestowed a great honor on him. He takes superior care of his pregnant women and their babies. Although famous as a pioneer in the childbirth world, Dr. Odent is also a lecturer and author of many books on child-birth and health.

Prior to his work in London, Odent helped women birth at the Centre Hospitalier General de Pithiviers, a public hospital about 50 miles south of Paris. He arrived at Pithiviers in 1962 to direct a surgical unit. At that time, many of the small French towns were in need of an ob-stetrician, and Odent, being a surgeon, was called by the midwives to perform C-sections or forceps deliveries. When the midwives kept put-ting women on their backs to deliver, Odent asked them why they in-sisted women birth this way. Their answer was because this is how they learned it in school. While on military duty in Algeria, Odent dealt with the war casualties in the hospitals, but he was also able to watch some of the local women giving birth according to local customs. After his service, he went to Africa and observed the struggle between the local women and the European-trained midwives who tried to make the women give birth in the recumbent position, instead of allowing them to squat in their traditional mode of birthing. This experience led Odent to begin questioning the Westernized system of assembly-line birth.

In Pithiviers Odent enabled women to labor in an unconventional manner. He had the labor rooms warmly decorated, consisting of car-peted platforms with big pillows. He also made warm pools of water available in case the women desired to use them. Use of the pools is neither suggested nor encouraged; they are there and can be used if that is what the woman wants or needs.

As it turned out, many women liked to labor in the pools and left the water when it was time to deliver the baby. Others, however, found the water to be of such comfort that they did not want to get out and chose to deliver their baby in the water. The newborns at this hospital are treated with the utmost care and respect, and they are not taken away from their mothers. Even premature babies are set in the rooms with their mothers, with the incubators right next to the bed.

Odent's attitude is one of care and respect for the birthing process. Women who are labeled high risk should be given even more respect so as not to disturb their intuitive decisions. Odent feels that the high-risk mother must not be fearful during labor, in order not to upset the hormonal balance, which could create problems in labor.

Dr. Odent practices anti-obstetrics, encouraging women to use their common sense in childbirth and to free themselves of the interventions that seem to pervade the medical philosophy of birth. Through his work, he has encouraged women to seek out new avenues in pregnancy and birth. When I asked one new mother, who read profusely during her pregnancy, to name the best book she had read during her preg-nancy, she at once replied: Odent's *Birth Reborn*.

THE U.S. INFLUENCE

By the early 1980s underwater birthing had become popular in many parts of the world. In 1980 in the United States, Patrick and Jia Lighthouse pioneered the way when they gave birth to Jeremy in the water in their home in Southern California. After hearing of their experience and the work of Odent and Charkowsky, others soon followed.

In the early 1980s I attended births throughout the San Francisco Bay area, and I soon began getting calls to help women with water births in Hawaii. Couples started coming from other states and staying with friends who lived in the Bay Area, so that they could have my assistance in helping their babies be born in water. At that time, little information was available on water births, and I was aware of no other birth practitioners who were willing to supply information and support women in their choice to labor and deliver as they chose.

In 1982, while at the Rainbow Dolphin Center in Tutukaka, New Zealand, where the First International Underwater Birth Conference was held, I ran into Phyllis Glickstein, a midwife from Portland, Oregon, who had attended several water births. She was also making pioneering efforts to support women in choosing a water birth in her community. She eventually moved to Detroit, where she now practices as a physician's assistant. Today Dr. Robert Doughton, who attended many water births in Portland, Oregon, can be used as a referral for the Portland area.

As of June 1993, water births were popular in most areas of the world. Most states in the United States have reported women laboring in water or actually giving birth in water. Occasionally, it may be difficult to find a midwife who will attend a water birth at home, but in states such as Massachusetts, New York, Michigan, Washington, Hawaii, Oregon, California, Nevada, New Mexico, and Alaska water births are well accepted.

Many more areas are making this opportunity available for women. Chris Griscom, for example, gave birth in the sea somewhere in the Bahamas, while another woman gave birth in a child's wading pool in San Juan, Puerto Rico. In 1987 Dr. Jan-Erik Strole, a Swedish obstetrician, attended a water birth at St. Joseph's Hospital in Polsen, Montana. After that birth, a few more water births took place in the hospital.

I am not aware of any hospitals in the United States, except the Family Birthing Center in Upland, California, where women can give birth in water. This center possesses some of the emergency resources found in a hospital. Women should be able to have the choice of using water in the hospitals, even if it is just for labor. Some women prefer to give birth in the hospital, but because of their affinity with water, they will birth at home. One problem yet to be overcome is that the insurance companies and hospitals are afraid of infections and other complications. This situation may change as more and more doctors and midwives throughout the world are supporting women's rights to have access to labor tanks.

INFLUENCES FROM OTHER PARTS OF THE WORLD

Many hospitals and birthing centers in Europe are making tanks available not only for labor but also for birthing. Many European countries have accepted the water milieu as a wonderful alternative to drug intervention. Fewer complications occur among women laboring in water then among those who have been administered drugs while in labor. As is well known, receiving drugs in labor can be a slippery slope leading to complications for both newborn and mother.

In England over one thousand women have labored and given birth in water to date. Sheila Kitzinger, a natural childbirth advocate, an anthropologist, and the author of numerous books on childbirth, has a grandchild who was born in water. Janet Balaskas, author of the books *New Active Birth* (1993) and *Water Birth* (1990), was inspired by her labor and delivery in water to write *Water Birth*. British hospitals are recognizing how the simple but marvelous qualities of water help laboring women. A few hospitals are actually installing tanks on their premises.

In Scandinavia, midwives and doctors are attending water births in both the home and the hospital. Hospitals in Stockholm, Sweden, and in Copenhagen, Denmark, have done research on labor and delivery in the water and have found favorable results. Suzanne Houd, a midwife in Copenhagen, is a contact for water births.

The beautiful seaport town of Oostende, Belgium, runs ferries back and forth to England. Dr. Hermann Ponnett, an obstetrician, works in a local hospital in the seaport town of Oostende, Belgium, where he bought his own tank for women to use while laboring and giving birth. The hospital liked the results so much that it bought him an even more elaborate tank and made it permanently available for women's use while in the hospital. Late one summer's evening Dr. Ponnett took me to the hospital. The doctor flicked on the lights and proudly displayed his beautiful tank. He said he had no problems with water births and would even do vacuum extractions under water. He stated that he only did the extractions if absolutely necessary and that performing them in water seemed to be easier on both mother and baby.

Outside of Brussels, near Waterloo, is a small country hospital where Dr. Serge Wesel serves as head obstetrician. The hospital allows women to labor in water, though not to give birth in this medium. Dr.

Wesel, inspired by the work of Dr. Odent, has been providing this service since the early 1980s. The labor room is comfortable, with a European-sized red bathtub. Nearby is a bed with pillows that hide the emergency equipment. Because Dr. Wesel does not feel comfortable with babies being born into the water, when it is time to start pushing, the mother gets out of the tank and delivers on the bed nearby.

Spain, too, has a hospital that offers water for labor and delivery, but most of the water deliveries have been done at home.

In 1989 an Italian woman visited me with plans she had designed for a birthing center in Rome that was to include a water-birthing room. Her plans seemed to rival the ancient Roman baths. I haven't heard from her lately, but perhaps the center is finished by now.

German women, as nearly all Western women, are concerned about good birthing practices. Methods associated with alternative medicine in the United States—homeopathy, herbs, Bach flower remedies—is part of German culture. Childbirth with a midwife is the norm in Germany, not the exception as it is here. Doctors, unless they are obstetricians, are required to ask a midwife to accompany them at a birth. Water labor and delivery is slowly being accepted, especially in Berlin. While in Berlin, I taught the water method in the Berlin Midwifery School and at the childbirth clinic of Maureen Amonis. At her clinic, Amonis has a beautiful birthing tank that resembles a giant bathtub. She feels very comfortable with water labor and delivery.

Midwife Suzanne Kuhnel in Munich, Germany, also attends water births at home. She has attended many such births and has also worked closely with Charkowsky. She reports the growing popularity of water births throughout Germany.

While speaking at the International Society of Pre- and Perinatal Psychology and Medicine Conference in Jerusalem in 1989, I met several Israeli midwives. Homebirths are illegal in Israel. Thus, when I did meet a couple who had a home water birth with a midwife, they would not disclose her name.

At the previously mentioned Maternity Unit in Pithiviers, France, women are able to use water for both labor and delivery. A couple I know from Berlin, Germany, went to Pithiviers and were very pleased with their midwives and their birth, stating that they had a beautiful experience. They reported, however, that fewer water births have taken place since Dr. Odent went to London.

Meloma Balaskas, who helped organize the Active Birth Movement in London, now lives in Capetown, South Africa, her native land. She returned there after a twenty-year absence and found that her help was needed in the childbirth world. She reports that many water births are occurring in South Africa, especially in Capetown.

In the early 1980s the Rainbow Dolphin Center in Tutukaka, New Zealand, was formed by water birth advocate Estelle Meyers to serve women who wanted to give birth in water. Many water births, assisted by midwives, have taken place at this center. Meyers has been instrumental in bringing international attention to water birthing and in establishing a networking system for those involved and interested in this approach to birth. Dr. Kamayani of Auckland, is on the board of the WATER organization, and can be contacted for information regarding water births in New Zealand.

Australia, a land filled with beautiful beaches and warm waters, has reportedly been the setting of numerous water births, especially in the seas of Monkey Mia. The reports also mention the presence of many dolphins in this area, which may be one reason for the attractiveness of the location. Many midwives attend water births in most other parts of Australia as well.

In 1989 I was interviewed by a Japanese film company that was making a movie about dolphins and whales in an effort to put a halt to the whaling industry in Japan. They included a water birth in their film, making the point that humans can give birth in water just as the cetaceans do. Since the showing of this film, water births have become increasingly popular in Japan.

Thus, as this brief summary indicates, humankind is finally realizing the great benefits of water births. People from all over the world are having water births, including new age enthusiasts, doctors, lawyers, chiropractors, and even a captain of a research vessel with whom I sailed. In the past thirteen years in the United States, the number of water births has increased steadily. It has gone past the point where it can be called "some new birthing fad." The Europeans have leaped ahead of the Americans, with more and more physicians and midwives singing water's praises for labor and delivery.

With the increasing number of research studies being conducted, laboring and giving birth in water is proving itself a healthy alternative to the ritualistic, interventive equipment and machines that have become so prevalent in the obstetric world. This intervention has made childbirth an unnatural event and, at times, unsafe for mother and baby.

Water birth has come a long way since Charkowsky's work in the 1960s. It gained popularity in the rest of the world in the early 1980s and by the early 1990s, laboring in water had become accepted by many practitioners in most parts of the world. At the same time, the benefits of water birth for the newborn are now being recognized. We need not so readily resort to pharmacological intervention when water brings safer, more satisfying results.

NOTES

1. The Human Relations Area Files, Inc. (HRAF) is an international research organization in the field of cultural anthropology. It is based at Yale University.

2. Donald Stanley Marshall, "Cuna Folk: A Conceptual Scheme involving the Dynamic Factors of Culture, as applied to the Cuna Indians of Darien." Unpublished manuscript, 1950. Included in the Human Relations Area Files, Yale University.

3. Marvel Elya Iglesias and Cristine Hudgins Morgan, "From the Cradle to the Grave: The Story of a Typical San Blas Indian Maiden." Cristobal, 1939. Included in the Human Relations Area Files, Yale University.

4. "A Water Birth in 1805," *Les Annales de la Société de Médecine Pratique de Montpellier* 5(13): 185–91.

5. Quote of Igor Charkowsky from audiotapes and notes that I made while working with him in Moscow and the Black Sea area.

6. Ibid.

7. Ibid.

8. Quote from an unpublished paper written by Igor Smirnov.

9. Ibid.

10. Ibid.

11. Quote of Igor Charkowsky from audiotapes and notes that I made while working with him in Moscow and the Black Sea area.

12. Ibid.

13. Ibid.

14. Ibid.

15. Ibid.

16. Ibid.

2

BIRTHING OPTIONS

In the last two decades new options in childbirth have become available, creating far greater choice for women than was possible only twenty years ago. More and more prospective parents are educating themselves as to their possible options. Both informed decisions and some soul searching are in order. Parents now must do some research of their own to answer an increasing number of questions: Where do I want to give birth? Is this really the best method for me and my baby? Where will I be the most comfortable and relaxed? Has my pregnancy had complications, or has it been uneventful, and how does that affect my choices? Do I want a doctor or a midwife to give me prenatal care and to attend my birth? Will the father of the newborn be able to catch (deliver) the baby?

Experiencing the birth of one's child is one of the most important and memorable events in anyone's life. When I speak of my occupation as a midwife, inevitably a passionate conversation will follow. Whether a man or a woman is involved, if a person has been present at a birth, especially the birth of his or her own child, the story will be told with much fervor.

Too often, women describe the births of their children with a tone of dissatisfaction. Most of these women lament, for example, about having to undergo caesarean sections, about being too drugged to bond with the baby, or about being unable to hold or nurse their baby because the baby was kept in the nursery. Women in these situations uniformly feel helpless and powerless. Researching one's options will help to empower couples to make the right decisions and to feel fulfilled after the momentous occasion of childbirth. This chapter describes all the choices that are presently available to women, especially in the West.

HOSPITAL BIRTHS

Since time began, women have been giving birth at home with a midwife in attendance. In the past fifty to sixty years, however, almost all women have been having their babies in hospitals. Why did this change take place?

For women with worries and concerns, the hospital setting may provide a greater sense of security. Women who are informed of complications during their pregnancies may feel safer giving birth in a place with emergency equipment that is quickly and easily obtained if necessary for both herself and her baby. The hospital setting also has many different personnel to take care of the laboring mother, as opposed to the one-on-one care of the traditional midwife.

Other women go to the hospital simply because it is the "thing to do," it is expected of her; after all, her mother and *her* mother before her gave birth in a hospital. An interesting corollary to this rationale was brought home to me during my travels in rural Denmark. There I met a woman who gave birth to her baby at home because her foremothers did. This was her tradition, and she thought it silly and extravagant to do anything else. It seemed strange to her that anyone would want to give birth any other way and especially not around a bunch of strangers.

Routine procedures conducted in hospitals, such as fetal heart monitoring, require the mother to lie still with a strap across her abdomen and an electrode inserted into the baby's scalp. The electrode cannot be placed in the baby's scalp unless the amniotic sac is broken. If this has not occurred naturally, then the amniotic sac must be artificially ruptured. According to some schools of thought, artificially rupturing the sac may do more harm than good and may cause serious complications for mother and baby.

Another standard hospital procedure is the insertion of a needle (IV) into the laboring mother's vein. This precautionary measure prepares the mother for surgery, prevents dehydration, and gives nourishment. Many women find this procedure restricting and uncomfortable, especially when they desire a natural childbirth with its consequent freedom of movement. The IV is used especially to induce labor with oxytocin and to prepare for doing a caesarean section (C-section or CSEC).

Because of the high rate of C-sections in the United States (25 to 30 percent), women are becoming more concerned about being able to labor in the manner they choose, let alone being able to give birth vaginally. Mothers are becoming more and more concerned for their own well-being and that of their newborn. Parents and professionals alike are asking why the CSEC rate has reached epidemic proportions in the last twenty years.

The World Health Organization recognizes the ramifications of the ever increasing use of invasive technology in birth. Many times the routine use of technology during labor leads to a domino effect involving other technologies. Interfering with and mistrusting nature, giving scientific materialism priority over common sense, can lead to more problems than it solves. The increased use of technology in the birth arena may well have contributed to the rise of the CSEC rate.

The CSEC rate has also risen in response to the threat of malpractice suits. As is well known, Americans have become a litigious people. Sometimes the suits are absolutely necessary, but at too many other times people are simply looking to make a quick and easy dollar. In reaction, the doctors seek to cover themselves by performing a CSEC in the event of complications and the birth of a less than "perfect" baby. The doctors, fearing the loss of their licenses, want to avoid court battles.

The long-established principle of "once a caesarean, always a caesarean" has also contributed to the rise in CSEC rates. This cry originated in the fear of uterine rupture in the event of a vaginal birth following a caesarean birth. In their well-researched book *Silent Knife* (1983), Nancy Wainer Cohen and Lois J. Estner state that in a lower segment incision (a transverse incision in the lower uterine segment), there is a 0.5 percent chance of uterine rupture in subsequent deliveries. Because of this small percentage, thousands have unnecessarily gone under the knife. In fact, Cohen and Estner believe that the term *rupture* is a serious misnomer. The term brings to mind life-threatening, catastrophic explosions, but these are extremely rare. More descriptive terms would be *separations, windows,* or *dehiscences,* which doctors sometimes find have occurred a week or two ahead of time while they are performing a repeat caesarean. Through Cohen and Estner's research, they found that rupture would produce a 0.1 percent maternal mortality. That is, there would be one maternal death out of 400,000 women. This is a much lower rate than the maternal deaths from a CSEC, which is 593 deaths out of 100,000 women. For those whom a caesarean section is a possibility, I strongly recommend reading *Silent Knife*.

Increasingly, some parents and professionals have come to believe that a CSEC produces less stress for the mother and baby. Occasionally, a prospective mother will tell me that she just wants to "get drugged up and get it cut out. Why should I go through all that pain?" When I speak with them after the operation, all they talk about is their post-surgical pain and how their healing took weeks and sometimes months. They also dwell on the "mean" nurses who made them walk around a day after their surgery, not realizing the nurses were doing this for their own good. What a contrast to the mother who has given birth at home, who is able to get out of bed with energy and enthusiasm. For post-CSEC mothers, lack of physical contact with their baby and the postponed breastfeeding were just as painful as their sutures. "I was too drugged up, and they wouldn't bring him to me for fear that I would drop him." Some of the women who thought they were getting off easy by having a CSEC describe their emotional pain with more intensity and sorrow than their physical pain.

CSEC babies are often described as beautiful, perfect-looking babies—maybe so, although beauty is in the eyes of the beholder. Some people have gotten a bit presumptuous with the theory that the infant is less stressed if artificially removed from the mother by a surgical procedure, rather than if nature is allowed to take its course by squeezing the baby out through the birth canal. Current research strongly affirms that the stress of the journey down the birth canal is absolutely necessary for a healthy newborn. In their article in the *Scientific American* (1986), Hugo Lagercrantz and Theodore A. Slotkin emphasize the importance of catecholamines for the survival of the newborn. These hormones are released during the "stress" of the journey through the birth canal. The authors suggest that the compression of the head in the birth canal greatly contributes to the release of the catecholamines and that the levels of these hormones were a lot lower in the infants born through elective CSEC without any labor.

These hormones help maintain the newborn's body, even though the newborn may be suffering oxygen deprivation. They increase the blood flow to the vital organs, such as the lungs and the heart, and send less to the extremities. Babies born vaginally are found to be more alert, thus possibly enhancing maternal–infant bonding.

Breech presentations have become another reason for a CSEC. (A breech presentation occurs when the baby's buttocks or feet, instead of the head, are in the downward position.) In medical schools today, many doctors are not being trained to deliver breech babies vaginally, but rather through caesarean sections, which are presumed to be safer. Therefore, vaginal breech births have become a lost art. A few "well-seasoned" doctors will attempt a breech vaginally if the conditions are right, such as when the mother's pelvis can accommodate the size of the baby's head. One high-risk perinatologist, after assisting a woman with a vaginal breech birth, told me, "This is more fun, CSECs are boring!"

A final factor in the increased CSEC rate is the doctor's pocketbook. I shudder to think that economics could be an incentive for a surgical procedure, but with the rate of CSECs up to 35 to 40 percent of all births in some California hospitals and the cost for the procedure as much as three times that of a vaginal birth, many people are wondering if the economic incentive isn't carrying too much weight.

Before giving birth, all prospective parents should interview their doctor and his or her associates and find out what their standards for birth are and especially their CSEC rates. The World Health Organization has recommended lowering the CSEC rates at least 10 percent. One can also investigate the physician's or hospital's CSEC rates by inquiring at the State Medical Association. The nurses on the obstetrical floor may also be able to give information.

Once the doctor is chosen, he or she should make a firm commitment to be at the birth—the laboring mother, expecting to see her own doctor at the time of her delivery, may be dismayed when one of her doctor's colleagues arrives instead as she is pushing her baby out. If she is not comfortable with this doctor, she may become distressed. In other instances, her doctor may be very busy and may arrive at the last minute. Thank God for the nurses who have breathed with her to help her stop pushing until the doctor arrives to deliver the baby.

Many pioneering parents, midwives, and doctors are successfully attempting vaginal births after a caesarean (VBACs) in the home and at the hospital. Several American midwives have reported excellent results with VBACs in warm water. As is true of any labor in water, VBAC women can relax better and dilate more easily. Contractions are more efficient in water, perhaps because of the water's warmth, which has a stimulating effect, helping the blood vessels to nourish the uterine and abdominal areas. VBACs laboring in water would be a worthwhile study, especially since it brings such good results for mothers.

In 1993 the Centers for Disease Control and Prevention reported that in 1991 doctors in the United States performed *349,000 unnecessary caesarean sections, which cost the nation more than $1 billion.* Of the 966,000 C-sections performed in the United States in 1991, 35 percent were repeats. The overall C-section rate was 23.5 per 100 births. Brazil and Puerto Rico were the only countries that reported higher rates. The report goes on to say that at one time C-sections were rare; by 1975 the rate was 10.4 per 100 births, and it rose to 24.7 births for every 100 in 1988. By the early 1990s it had risen even higher. The number of VBAC deliveries is also increasing, however. The study showed that 108,000 women (24.2 births per 100 deliveries) delivered vaginally in 1991 after a previous C-section. In 1990 the average was only 20.4 births out of 100. In some ways this study is very encouraging. VBAC women need support in their desire to have vaginal deliveries. In this regard, labor and delivery in water is a successful way to help women to relax, enabling a vaginal delivery to occur.

Precisely where the mother delivers her baby can be problematic in a hospital. Many mothers want to give birth in the room where they labored and don't want to have to be transferred to a delivery room when it is time to push out the baby. Most hospitals, however, insist that the "procedure" take place in a delivery room where more of the emergency equipment is immediately on hand. This equipment can be life saving, such as in cases of hemorrhage, failure to push the baby out, forceps, vacuum extraction, emergency caesarean sections, resuscitation of the newborn, or a full-on neonatal team. Indeed, complications may arise, but 95 percent of the time childbirth is uneventful.

Depending on the circumstances of the birth and the doctor's philosophy, the baby may go directly onto the mother's breast, or hospital policies may demand that the baby go to the nursery to be looked over and observed.

Some couples object to their babies being whisked off to the nursery and left there. In most states procedures such as PKU, vitamin K, erythromycin emollient in the baby's eyes, and the examination of the newborn are routinely done on the baby and are the law. Parents may sign a form declining the administration of these drugs, but before doing so, they should consult a health care provider. It is important to research this issue ahead of time, getting all the information possible. A few parents request that all the procedures be done in the same room where the mother gave birth. Some are able to hold their baby while the procedures are taking place, enabling them to comfort the baby afterward. This is a perfect time for the man to do his fathering while the mother is resting.

Circumcision of male babies is also fairly standard in American hospitals. In this surgical procedure, the foreskin of the penis is removed and often with no anesthetic. Thus, the baby experiences pain while the procedure is being done. It leaves the penis swollen and red, and extremely painful for days. The doctors need the parents' approval before performing this procedure. Some parents see no reason for it and leave their boys' God-given piece of skin intact.

By 1994 one would hope that all hospitals allow fathers to be present at the birth of their babies. Of course, much depends on how involved the father wants to be. One father told me of his gratifying experience in a hospital in Oakland, California. He and his wife planned a homebirth, but when last-minute complications arose, she was transported by ambulance to the hospital. The father was able to catch (receive) his baby, cut the umbilical cord, and hold the baby while the mother was delivering the placenta. Since there were no severe complications, his request for maximum participation was encouraged.

Although in the United States and a few European countries the trend has been toward giving birth in hospitals, no study has ever proven that hospital births are safer than homebirths. In fact, statistics from the World Health Organization bring up questions as to the safety and efficacy of modern childbirth technology. The Netherlands, where most women have their babies at home, has the fifth lowest infant mortality rate in the Western world, while the United States ranks a woeful twenty-fourth. Significantly, the United States has proportionally fewer homebirths and is just starting to use midwives again.

Most women have been taught to fear pregnancy and birth. From youth on, "Women and children die in childbirth," echoes in our ears. In their book *Lying In,* (1977), Richard and Dorothy Wertz state:

> Even if all the women in seventeenth-century Plymouth who died during childbearing years died because of birth complications, birth was still successful 95% of the time. Since many of these women must have died of infections or other diseases, colonial birth, while dangerous and fearful, was still not quite the calamity moderns picture it to have been (p. 12).

The book shows that nutritional and environmental factors were of great importance for the mother's health and longevity, depending on whether they had a sufficent amount of food and decent housing. The Wertzes also reveal that women of lower economic status had to return to their household chores immediately, for hungry mouths could not wait—nor could work in the fields be postponed long.

Wertz and Wertz also state that

> Some historians have estimated (colonial) infants' deaths in early months to be as high as 10%. Many infants died, however, because of infectious diseases rather than birth damage—Children in American seaport towns, however, had less chance for longevity than children in American farming communities, for infections were more prevalent along the coasts (p. 12).

Women need an atmosphere where they are encouraged to labor and give birth in the way they feel is the best. Feeling secure and safe is an important contributing factor to easier labor and delivery. Hospitals and their staff may or may not be able to provide this kind of security. Getting educated as to what one wants and needs can help the mother make an informed decision. After all, she is not under arrest, and she can make her decisions with the help of her partner or birth advocate. Birth in a hospital can be a fullfilling experience, free from unnecessary interventions if her desires and needs are discussed ahead of time.

All pregnant women should study the "Pregnant Patient's Bill of Rights" endorsed by the International Childbirth Education Association (ICEA). (It is reprinted here with permission of the International Childbirth Education Association, © International Childbirth Education Association, Minneapolis, Minnesota 55420 USA.) These rights are as follows:

1. The Pregnant Patient has the right, prior to the administration of any drug or procedure, to be informed by the health professional caring for her of any potential direct or indirect effects, risks, or hazards to herself or her unborn or newborn infant which may result from the use of a drug or procedure prescribed for or administered to her during pregnancy, labor, birth, or lactation.

2. The Pregnant Patient has the right, prior to the proposed therapy, to be informed, not only of the benefits, risks, and hazards of the proposed therapy but also of known alternative therapy, such as available childbirth education classes which could help to prepare the Pregnant Patient physically and mentally to cope with the discomfort or stress of pregnancy and the experience of childbirth, thereby reducing or eliminating her need for drugs and obstetric intervention. She should be offered such information early in her pregnancy in order that she may make a reasoned decision.

3. The Pregnant Patient has the right, prior to the administration of any drug, to be informed by the health professional who is prescribing or administering the drug to her that any drug which she receives during pregnancy, labor and birth, no matter how or when the drug is taken or administered, may adversely affect her unborn baby, directly or indirectly, and that there is no drug or chemical which has been proven safe for the unborn child.

4. The Pregnant Patient has the right if caesarean section is anticipated, to be informed prior to the administration of any drug, and preferably prior to her hospitalization, that minimizing her, and in turn, her baby's intake of nonessential pre-operative medicine will benefit her baby.

5. The Pregnant Patient has the right, prior to the administration of a drug or procedure, to be informed of the areas of uncertainty if there is *no* properly controlled follow-up research which has established the safety of the drug or procedure with regard to its direct and/or indirect effects on the physiological, mental and neurological development of the child exposed, via the mother, to the drug or procedure during pregnancy, labor, birth, or lactation—(this would apply to virtually all drugs and the vast majority of obstetric procedures).

6. The Pregnant Patient has the right, prior to the administration of any drug, to be informed of the brand name and generic name of the drug in order that she may advise the health professional of any past adverse reaction to the drug.

7. The Pregnant Patient has the right to determine for herself, without pressure from her attendant, whether she will accept the risks inherent in the proposed therapy or refuse a drug or procedure.

8. The Pregnant Patient has the right to know the name and qualifications of the individual administering a medication or procedure to her during labor or birth.

9. The Pregnant Patient has the right to be informed, prior to the administration of any procedure, whether that procedure is being administered to her for her or her baby's benefit (medically indicated) or as elective procedure (for convenience, teaching purposes or research).

10. The Pregnant Patient has the right to be accompanied during the stress of labor and birth by someone she cares for and to whom she looks for emotional comfort and encouragement.

11. The Pregnant Patient has the right after appropriate medical consultation to choose a position for labor and for birth which is least stressful to her baby and to herself.

12. The Obstetric Patient has the right to her baby cared for at her bedside if her baby is normal, and to feed her baby according to her baby's needs rather than according to the hospital regimen.

13. The Obstetric Patient has the right to be informed in writing of the name of the person who actually delivered her baby and the professional qualifications of that person. This information should also be on the birth certificate.

14. The Obstetric Patient has the right to be informed if there is any known or indicated aspect of her or her baby's care or condition which may cause her or her baby later difficulty or problems.

15. The Obstetric Patient has the right to have her and her baby's hospital medical records complete, accurate and legible and to have their records, including Nurses' Notes, retained by the hospital until the child reaches at least the age of majority, or, alternatively, to have the records offered to her before they are destroyed.

16. The Obstetric Patient, both during and after her hospital stay, has the right to have access to her complete hospital medical records, including Nurses' Notes, and to receive a copy upon payment of a reasonable fee and without incurring the expense of retaining an attorney.

Giving birth in a hospital can be a very fulfilling event. Many women relate how smoothly the labor and delivery went. They felt well taken care of, and their doctors and nurses were open to many of the couple's needs and desires. They also felt safe and secure. "I wouldn't have done it any other way," a new young mother told me. The common denominator among these women who felt good about their hospital births was that they went into the hospital knowing what they wanted and didn't want. Occasionally, some presented a list of demands to the doctor and the hospital staff sometime during the pregnancy. This list not only gives the doctor and staff an idea of what is wanted, but also helps to make the prospective parents think about what is important to them.

ALTERNATIVE BIRTH ROOM/CENTER (ABC)

Alternative birthing rooms are private rooms in hospitals designed to bring the comforts of home into the hospital. The room is usually decorated in a homey style, with curtains, stereo, and a double-sized bed that transforms into a delivery bed in case of an emergency. Emergency equipment is usually concealed behind a panel or curtain and is readily available. Couples have privacy and are able to give birth in the same room and bed. For some, the homelike setting, combined with the "security" of being in the hospital, is a comfort.

Mothers are carefully screened, and only low-risk mothers are able to use the alternative rooms. When these rooms are in great demand, they are, of course, not always available. Some hospitals book reservations, but it is always possible that another woman may be laboring in the room at the time you may need it.

Depending on the staff's standards and flexibility, the woman can move about as she pleases and may be supported to get into the delivery position that she intuitively feels is best. The father and the children may be able to take part in the event, but once again this may go against hospital policies.

Some obstetricians do not like to use the alternative birthing rooms because they feel it is more time consuming. Since some obstetricians have a heavy patient load, their services may not be as frequent as the laboring mothers would like them to be.

Several criticisms of the ABC rooms have been voiced. Some parents feel that a separate staff for the ABC should be available. Usually, however, the same hospital staff takes care of both high- and low-risk women. A nurse, for example, may be unavailable for monitoring and support owing to the needs of higher risk women with more problems. As a result, women with normally progressing labors who still need help and support may be left alone. A separate staff for the ABC room, with more flexible policies and regulations, would be more advantageous for the mother. For the attendants, the person may be one of many coming through the hospital, while for the mother, it will be a unique experience that she will remember for the rest of her life.

In an article in *Birth* (1983), Michael Klein wrote of the high transfer rates from the ABC to the delivery rooms. In his study he sent letters to 120 ABCs in North America. He received 30.8 percent replies. Of the facilities that responded, 44 percent allowed only minor procedures such as shaving, enema, local anesthesia, IV, fetal monitoring (external and internal), and repair of an episiotomy in their ABCs. However, 56 percent of the respondents permitted both minor and major procedures in their ABCs, including all the previously mentioned procedures as well as the use of oxytocin for stimulation or augmentation, artificially rupturing the amniotic sac, forceps, epidurals, vacuum extraction, twin delivery, delivery of a baby with meconium, and pre-eclampsia. He found that the highest transfer rates were among those in tertiary (university) hospitals and in the ABCs that only allowed minor procedures. His findings showed that the hospitals that had the fewest restrictions and regulations for women laboring and delivering in their ABC rooms had the lowest transfer rates to the delivery rooms and the lowest number of interventive measures taken.

Depending on the insurance company, most ABCs are covered by insurance policies. Some parents and professionals believe that one reason why hospitals install these rooms is to seduce couples who are vacillating between a home or a hospital setting to give birth in the hospital.

Again, careful screening of the policies regarding the ABC is to be encouraged. Look at the hospital statistics. What is the success rate of women able to give birth in the rooms? Occasionally, mothers have been disappointed with the experience as a whole when having a birth in an ABC, because they were told they would have something they didn't get. Others have been very pleased with their experiences.

OUT-OF-HOSPITAL OR FREESTANDING BIRTH CLINICS

Freestanding birthing centers/clinics are separate from the hospital. They are different around the world, differing in the length of time the mother is required to stay, ranging from a few hours to a few days. For some the birthing clinics/centers are the best of both worlds, that is, hospital and home. Mothers feel comfortable because they are able to give birth in the bed in which they have labored. The family and support team can also be present. Barring complications, the newborn can usually stay with the mother after the birth. Intervention may be minimal, but screening of the center's policies is advised. Depending on the insurance company and state, the cost of these birth centers may be covered.

I visited such a center for a few months in 1990 as a guest midwife in a birth center in Berlin, Germany. The center was owned and operated by a German midwife who was seeing several women who wanted to have water births. Since there was little information about water births in Berlin, let alone about someone who was experienced in attending such births, I was brought in from California to teach midwives and help with the deliveries.

I was very impressed with the birth center, which was a large flat in

one of the main sections of Berlin. The flat had several large rooms—
two large rooms for childbirth classes and exercises, an office, a waiting
room, a kitchen, a beautiful large room for labor and delivery, and, most
interesting to me, a large bathroom with a bath big enough for three.
The mothers could comfortably move around in the bath, which was
deep enough for them to get into a squatting position. The fathers were
also delighted to be able to get into the bath and catch their own babies.
Although the labor-bed was just a few feet down the hall, we found it
necessary to put a mat next to the bath if the mother had an emergency
and had to get out of the bath quickly.

The center employed five midwives. Each couple had their own midwife with whom they had worked throughout the pregnancy. This
proved a comfort for the pregnant mothers because they knew this same
midwife would be there with them at the delivery of their babies. All
the midwives were excited to learn about water births and encouraged
the women to use the warm water to help with the delivery.

Europe has many freestanding birthing centers. It is quite common
for Europeans to have their babies in a clinic. More and more hospitals
and clinics are also making water available for women to labor and give
birth in.

At this writing, just one birth center in the United States allows
women to give birth in water. This is the Family Birthing Center of
Upland, California. As of 1989, 483 births have occurred there in water,
all with good outcomes. Through this clinic's pioneering efforts, more
centers in the United States will be offering water for laboring women.

A lot depends on the clinics' policies, the doctors, and the staff. Before
making any final decisions, it is best to "shop around" to find out what
feels best for all involved.

HOMEBIRTHS

My introduction to homebirth was through a dear friend who wanted
my comfort and support at the birth of her child in her home in the
mountains of the high desert in Southern California. Jane lived miles
back in the mountains, a journey of almost an hour on rocky dirt roads.
I wondered to myself why she would choose the "risk" of staying at
home. At that time all my medical experience consisted of work in physical therapy and occupational therapy in hospitals. (This was prior to
my training as a midwife.) My background had left me with a fear that
the human body could not perform properly unless under the direction
of a doctor with access to all the latest medical technology.

Because of my deep respect for my friend, I trusted her decision,
despite my trepidations, and I agreed to be there for her. Besides, as
she put it, "My other babies came quickly. I would never make it down

that mountain, and no doctor wants to come up that road in her Cadillac!"

Eventually, Jane went into labor, and her neighbor came to get me. Jane was smiling happily as I walked through the door. With her was her husband and a woman I had never met before—her midwife. I clenched my teeth, waiting for the hysterical woman to emerge. It never happened. She smiled between contractions. Her midwife was very competent, checking the baby's heartbeat, helping Jane's breathing, and giving her encouragement. Flashes of Hollywood movies filled my mind: women screaming out and carrying on during labor. The labor and delivery wards in the hospitals where I worked had echoed with screams for help, and no one seemed to know what to do for these women.

I wasn't much help at this birth. I was awestruck by my friend, who obviously had pain but seemed to handle it quite well. A few hours later, she gave birth to an 8-pound baby girl. The baby snuffled a bit but wasn't screaming with terror like the newborns I had viewed through the glass at the hospital nurseries. The baby looked around, settling her eyes on a bouquet of bright red flowers beside the bed. She seemed to concentrate her gaze on the flowers; then she closed her eyes and slept. "Babies can't see when they are so young," I said. Everyone just laughed at my ignorance. After an hour of sleep the baby nursed. Mother and baby were obviously well and happy.

What was apparent at my friend's birth was the trust Jane had in her body and in nature. She seemed to know what to do for herself to help the labor and delivery proceed in a healthy way. I was most impressed with the midwife who had all the skills and equipment necessary to help the process of labor as a harmonious, not a discordant, event. She, too, trusted the womanly process of birth enough to let nature take its course, intervening only if complications arose.

Many women are again turning to homebirths because of this trust in nature and in their bodies. A lot of women express concern about giving birth in hospitals, for fear of having to surrender their instinctive abilities to the technology and interventive measures of the hospital.

As noted earlier, statistics show that the United States has one of the highest infant mortality rates in the Western world, ranking number twenty-fourth out of twenty-seven countries. Most babies in the United States are born in the hospital with a doctor in attendance, while in the Netherlands, which ranks in the top five (the lower end of infant mortality), most babies are born at home with midwives. Majorie Tew, a medical research statistician, researched the national perinatal statistics for Holland, which were taken in 1986. In a journal called *Midwifery* she states: "In births after 32 weeks gestation, the mortality is much lower under the noninterventionist care of midwives than under the interventionist management of obstetricians at all levels of predicted risk" (1990, p. 64). In the same journal, studies showed that "At gestations of 33–36 weeks the perinatal mortality rate (PNMR) was very significantly higher for obstetricians (46.4) than for midwives (12.6). . . . At gestations greater than 36 weeks, 93.3% of total births and nearly half of them under obstetricians' care, the perinatal mortality rate was ten times higher for obstetricians (8.1) than for midwives (0.8)" (p. 64). The Dutch study shows that after 32 weeks, 98.2 percent of the babies born have a 12 percent lower mortality (PNMR 1.0) if put under a midwife's care in the home or in the hospital, as opposed to being put under an obstetrician's care in the hospital (PNMR 11.9)

Obstetricians have forced midwifery out of the childbirth world for many decades in the United States. During the late 1960s the women's movement brought about a new awareness of women's responsibilities for their own bodies. Women began to demand more control over their own reproductive processes, and they also wanted to revive the old tradition of women taking care of women—midwives. It is one of the occupations unique to women that has fallen by the wayside.

Women found they could have greater control if they gave birth at home. This resulted in a resurgence of midwifery since few doctors would attend a homebirth. Women choosing midwives found that they were receiving superior prenatal care, as well as having the comfort of the midwife's womanly care during labor, delivery, and the postpartum period—all in the comfort of their own home.

Some, lacking knowledge and information, fear home birth. Certainly, if serious complications should arise in the pregnancy, a hospital birth may be essential. One of my main guiding principles on this subject is that the mother should give birth wherever she feels most comfortable, for this level of comfort will help her to relax and labor and delivery can then progress with greater ease.

Yet another philosophy is involved here: the technological philosophy. This way of thinking holds that the greater use of technology and specialists produces better outcomes. This philosophy is, of course, utilized in the hospital. But of all the studies comparing home and hospital births, "hospital births have never been proven to have better outcomes or were safer," says Dr. M. Wagner, head of the Maternal and Infant Division, World Health Organization.

The homebirth philosophy is part not only of the feminist revolution, but also of the health revolution in self-care. People want to take more responsibility for their own health care and do not want to surrender it entirely to professionals. They seek professional help for diagnosis, advice, and information, not for orders or scare tactics. Usually, people who want homebirths are not totally disavowing the hospitals and the specialists. Indeed, they realize the importance of their availability in an emergency situation. Instead, homebirth people simply want to take the responsibility to construct the kind of birth that will suit their needs. They look at pregnancy and childbirth not as a disease but as an act of nature.

Once the decision for a homebirth has been made, how does a person go about achieving it? Pregnant couples often find their birth attendant through word of mouth. Usually a friend has had a baby at home or knows of someone who has. In addition, a La Leche League leader is generally listed in the telephone book. This organization is dedicated to providing information and support on breastfeeding and usually also has current information on midwives and doctors who will attend a homebirth.

Once a doctor or a midwife has been located, it is important to interview the person to find out if he or she agrees with the pregnant woman's philosophies, and is someone the woman feels comfortable with as well as someone she will want to share one of the most miraculous times in her life. It is also important for the pregnant mother to trust that her doctor or midwife will be supportive of her needs while in labor and be capable of handling any emergency situation so that she can relax and let her body work as it needs to in order to give birth to her baby.

When interviewing a midwife, some of the following questions may help you decide whether or not to engage this person.

1. *Where did the midwife receive her training, and with whom did she train?*

If you have choices between a certified nurse midwife (CNM) and a traditional midwife (also known as a lay or direct entry midwife), you are very fortunate to have the opportunity to be able to make a choice. What is important is that the midwife evoke the feeling of supporting the pregnant woman in trusting in her own body, that the midwife herself knows how to trust in the womanly function of birth, and that she has enough confidence and wisdom in herself as a midwife to resist giving in to fear when a complication arises. Being able to keep a clear head and perform well in emergency situations is an extremely valuable tool.

2. *With what complications has she had hands-on experience?*

A midwife should have a current CPR certificate and be well versed in the resuscitation of a newborn. She should be able to identify any signs of complications or conditions during the labor that may endanger both the mother and the baby. Has the midwife ever handled a hemorrhaging mother? Has she handled a shoulder dystocia (a situation where the head of the baby is out of the mother's vagina and the shoulders get stuck)? What does she do for a retained placenta?

3. *At how many births has she been the primary caregiver? How many has she attended at home and how many in the hospital?*

The midwife and doctor under whom I apprenticed were not comfortable "kicking me out of the nest" until I had been the primary caregiver through fifty supervised pregnancies and fifty supervised labors and deliveries. I felt that these were necessary standards, for they gave me self-confidence and a broader perspective of pregnancy and birth. All in all, it put me out in the field as a qualified, skilled midwife.

4. *What is her philosophy about pregnancy and birth?*

Just as a few doctors carry around an "I am god" attitude, so, too, can a midwife. In my opinion, a birth attendant should be a "fly on the wall" during a labor, making suggestions and intervening only when absolutely necessary. If a birth attendant tries to control the labor, only complications can arise, because the birth attendant is then not empowering the mother to use her own instincts. Some birth attendants may come to a birth with an attitude about how the mother is *supposed* to labor, not how she *needs* to labor. If a mother senses this happening, she can lose all confidence in her ability to labor as only she knows how. It is important that the midwife's philosophies and approaches to birth be in accord with those of the mother's and father's.

5. *Will she be an active participant in the prenatal care?*

Occasionally, I will meet a midwife who doesn't do the prenatal care and instead depends on the backup doctor for this important function. I would steer clear of such a situation. Part of being a midwife is ensuring that a woman gets good prenatal care, and this means taking an active part in such aspects of care as nutritional counseling, educating the mother about pregnancy and birth, and monitoring the gestational changes that indicate fetal and maternal well-being, such as blood pressure, urine tests, fetal heartbeat, measuring the growth of the baby by measuring the growth of the mother's uterus (checking fundal height), watching the mother's weight, and periodically having blood work done. The midwife also needs to assess how the pregnant mother is doing emotionally, giving her help and support if necessary.

It is important to know how often the midwife will want to see you. In a pregnancy that proceeds normally—that is, a pregnancy that is not indicative of complications—it is standard for a mother to see her practitioner once a month until the eighth month of pregnancy. After that, the mother should see the midwife every two weeks until the ninth month, and then once a week until the baby is born.

6. Does she have doctor backup for consulting? Does she have a doctor who will meet the mother and her at the hospital if any complications occur during the labor?

It is equally important to meet the doctor with whom the midwife works. One of my mottoes concerning pregnancy and birth is "Be Prepared" to cover all bases. If you should need to go to the hospital during your labor, it is good to know the person who is going to take over under these new circumstances. This doctor should have supportive attitudes and the wisdom to let nature proceed, as long as the health of the mother and baby are not jeopardized.

7. If no doctor backup is available, what plan of action does she have in case of an emergency?

Unfortunately, it is becoming more and more difficult to find a doctor who supports couples who want a homebirth. Thus, it has become very hard to get a doctor to meet a couple in the hospital should complications arise. This leaves the midwife and the couple in labor out on a limb, with their only choice being to seek help in the emergency room of the local hospital. I do not feel good about this situation because the woman in labor will be taking a chance on what doctor she will get when she arrives at the hospital. The doctor may have an attitude about homebirth as well as those who attempt them. At any rate, in an emergency situation, lives may be at stake, and that is the bottom line.

More and more midwives, licensed or unlicensed, have had to resort to the emergency room in order to support the demands of their birthing community when doctor backup is unavailable. For various reasons, few doctors will attend homebirths, and most midwives will. If more people stick to their beliefs and principles and demand that doctors serve them as they want and need, perhaps these kinds of situations will not arise as often.

8. How soon does she go "on call" before the baby is due?

Being "on call" means that the midwife should be available and reachable two and one-half to three weeks before the baby's due date. For years I worked without an electronic pager and left telephone numbers of the places I could be reached. This made life difficult for me and somewhat for the pregnant couples as well, because it was sometimes hard to reach me. Although I never missed a birth, I still strongly advise getting your midwife a pager if she doesn't already have one. It puts the couples at ease to know they can reach the midwife at any time.

9. When does she come to the birth?

I am always very circumspect as to when I arrive at a birth. Timing is very important. I don't want to arrive too early and perhaps infringe on a very special bonding time for the couple. Nor do I want to arrive too late and not give the needed attention to the mother and baby, such as listening to the baby's heartbeat and assisting the mother with her labor—not to mention missing the birth entirely. I usually ask couples when they want me to arrive. I find that first-time moms need verification early on in labor that this is the real thing and not false labor. "Experienced" couples seem to want to have a bit of alone time before they give me a call.

10. *Will she bring an assistant?*

An assistant can be another midwife, an apprentice midwife, or a labor coach. I know very few midwives who will work alone. Working with another skilled midwife or apprentice is essential to good care. If an emergency situation occurs, it is better for both mother and baby to have extra hands than for one person to have to attend two people. A labor coach is valuable in helping the mother with her breathing, relieving the father, and assisting with the little but important things that need to be carried out at a birth. Unless the labor coach is experienced with complications at births, I cannot recommend her acting as a full assistant for the midwife.

11. *What equipment does she bring to the birth?*

Midwives should bring the basic equipment: a fetoscope or a doppler to listen to the baby's heartbeat; a blood pressure cuff and stethoscope for assessing the blood pressure; oxygen for the mother during labor or after, as well as for the newborn if problems with breathing arise. Some midwives will bring an ambu-bag for emergency resuscitation of the newborn, IV fluids for mothers who are unable to keep any fluids down and become dehydrated, medication to give the mother an injection to control a hemorrhage, herbs, and various other items.

12. *How long does she stay after the birth?*

After the placenta has been born, I feel it necessary to stay in the couple's home for approximately three hours. This is, of course, if there have been no complications for the mother or the newborn. In the event of complications, it is advisable to start counting the three hours after the complications have been brought under complete control and the mother and the baby are adjusting well.

13. *When does the midwife start her postpartum care?*

The midwife should return within the first twenty-four hours to make sure the mother and the baby are adapting well to breastfeeding. It is also advisable for the midwife to check the baby for jaundice, as well as noting urination and bowel movements. Estimating the amount of maternal bleeding is also part of postpartum care.

If the breastfeeding is going well and the other factors mentioned above are normal, the midwife may not have to come again until the third day after the baby is born for further followup. Contact by phone should be available and a six-week check up is advisable.

14. *What are her fees? Do her fees include payment for the assistant?*

Some midwives find it practical to break the fee up into categories—that is, prenatal care, assistant fee, birth attendance, and postpartum care. Some may charge more for extra prenatal and postpartum care. All these issues need to be discussed so that everything is absolutely up front and out in the open. Most midwives want to be paid in full before the birth; in this way they can protect themselves. Once the baby is born, the midwife can't put him back. It is easy for some couples to get caught up in the day-to-day bills. Heaven knows how quickly they fly in once the baby arrives, and so occasionally the midwife's fees get put on the bottom of the priority list.

Most medical insurance policies won't cover the midwife's fees. A few will cover certified nurse midwives, and, depending on the state, the government may cover the costs.

The most important factor to consider is, How comfortable do you feel with the midwife? Is this someone whom you want present at one of the most intimate times in your life? Will she support you to have the labor and birth that you want, or will she try to take over?

One couple whom I assisted at their water birth became pregnant again about a year after their "water baby" was born. Having had a wonderful experience with their first birth, they remarked that they would not have changed a thing. Money was scarce with this second pregnancy, but they did have health insurance. Even though I told them I trusted that they would pay me and told them I would take time payments, they decided in the end that they did not want to be saddled with payments and believed they could stand up for and get what they wanted in the hospital. Although they had a beautiful baby girl, they felt deprived of a potentially fulfilling experience. Later, they told me that no amount of money can be placed on a precious experience that happens only a few times in one's life. Unless the fee is far beyond one's means, it may be worth it to go into debt a bit, shoot for the stars, and get what every woman deserves—the fulfillment to give birth in the manner she wants. With this in mind, the parents must accept responsibility for the birth.

Even though a doctor or a midwife may be present, the mother and father are primarily responsible for what goes on during labor and delivery. No one can be expected to take over this responsibility. Only the individual involved has ultimate responsibility for making the final decisions to create the birth experience that she wants. When interviewing a doctor who is willing to attend a home delivery, I find the same questions that apply in interviewing a midwife useful. Some doctors can attend a homebirth and accept insurance.

The doctor with whom I apprenticed is a rare doctor indeed. While learning my art (midwifery), the senior midwife and I were the primary attendants for the laboring mother. The position he took was that of the "fly on the wall," trusting that the mother knew what to do and supporting the midwives in their decisions. I vividly recall a birth in which the doctor sat in the corner for most of the labor reading a gardening magazine, yet he was very much present and attentive to what was taking place in the labor. He was there if needed for an emergency, but he also respected the couple's need for intimacy. His presence was most nonintrusive. When the baby's head was born, we said, "Doctor, the baby is coming!" He looked up, smiled and said, "So I see." Standing to the side, he silently watched the delivery. His presence was very comforting for everyone there, not because he was a doctor or a man, but because he was so calm and relaxed. His relaxed, confident attitude set the tone in the room. It seemed to say, "Yes, here is an everyday natural occurrence. There is no reason to treat it any other way." This kind of equanimity is needed at every birth. If an emergency occurs, it is to be dealt with in the calmest manner possible. Panic only makes for chaos, which doesn't help the person in trouble.

WHO IS A GOOD CANDIDATE FOR A HOMEBIRTH?

A few practitioners I know consult the book, *Home Birth: A Practitioner's Guide,* which lists eligibility criteria for homebirth. By the standards of some doctors and midwives (and my own standards), it is a fairly conservative guide. While the individual's health and state of mind need to be taken into account, nonetheless these criteria should be considered. This list doesn't mean that the person who happens to fit into one of these categories should avoid a homebirth, especially if the person is in good physical and emotional health. When making a decision for the safety of one's baby and self, all factors, conservative or not, should be taken into account.

The following list is reprinted from *Home Birth: A Practitioner's Guide to Birth Outside the Hospital,* by S. E. Sagov, R. I. Feinbloom, P. Spindel, and A. Brodsky, pp. 69–70, with permission of Aspen Publishers, Inc., © 1984. The guide states the following contraindications to homebirths:

I. Contraindications to Planned Home Birth at Initial Screening

   A. Sociodemographic and logistical

1. Age

   a. Primipara (first time mother) below 18 or above 35

   b. Multipara (more than one baby) over 40

2. Distance from backup hospital too great (over 20 minutes driving time in average traffic)

3. Physical or emotional inadequacy of home environment as revealed by interviews and/or home visit

4. Unwillingness or incapacity to undertake prenatal education

B. Obstetric and medical history

   1. Preexisting chronic diseases (e.g., obesity, diabetes, hypertension, significant cardiac conditions) or emotional disturbances

   2. Grand multiparity (more than five previous births)

   3. Previous caesarean section

   4. Previous birth of a baby with serious congenital anomaly of a probably repeating type that cannot be excluded through antenatal evaluation

All these criteria warrant additional comments here.

To start with, in my opinion the age factor is sometimes used in an overly protective manner. It is true that women under 18 years of age may run a greater risk, but this is due mainly to the possibility of a not yet fully developed pelvis, lack of maturity, and an inadequate diet. Sometimes the typical teen diet may not be sufficiently well balanced to provide good nutrition for a body that is rapidly changing and to feed a developing fetus adequately. On the other hand, more teens are becoming conscious of eating right and are staying away from junk foods.

First-time mothers over 35 years of age may statistically have longer labors and have higher transfer rates (incidences of having to go to the hospital) while in labor, but I have not noticed this in my practice. The women over 35 whom I see are women who have been extremely well educated in nutrition and exercise. Many are healthier and more physically fit than many women in their twenties. They also have a good frame of mind about childbirth. By the time they reach this age, they have accomplished many things they have wanted to do. They are mature women who really want to be mothers, and they are ready to take on the responsibilities of motherhood.

As for women over 40 years of age who previously have had children, several things have to be ascertained before homebirth is contraindicated. How many previous pregnancies has the woman had? Were there complications in the previous pregnancies? Were the labors and deliveries uneventful? Again, nutrition and exercise are an important component in the pregnant woman's well-being. Will she be too stressed if she has more children?

When living in a rural area, the distance from the backup hospital may be greater than twenty minutes; this may be a risk the couple is willing to take. I have spoken with midwives living near Hudson Bay, working with indigenous families, who in some situations are a three-hour helicopter ride from the nearest hospital. If an emergency arises, it is crucial that the right equipment be already on hand. This is an admittedly extreme situation but a nonetheless real one in many parts of the world. In some parts of California, it may be an hour's drive to the closest hospital. The parents are ultimately responsible for the decision to stay at home, bearing in mind the possibility that they may have to drive to the hospital in a situation that could endanger the lives of both mother and baby. My friend Jane who lived far up in the mountains was afraid she wouldn't make it to the hospital on time if she attempted to get in the car and drive. Her fear was that she would have the baby on the side of the mountain road, which helped her decision to have a homebirth. To reiterate, ultimately it is the couple's responsibility to decide what is best for them. Their caregiver is there to help educate them to make a responsible decision.

With regard to the physical or emotional inadequacies of the home, the midwife must keep evaluating this factor throughout the pregnancy. If the house is filthy with animals running in and out, it may not be a healthy environment for a homebirth. If good water is not available, perhaps it is better to find an alternative setting or go to the hospital.

Just as important is the emotional situation. I can relate stories of women being emotionally abandoned by their husbands or partners and experiencing complications at the time of labor or delivery. Psychological problems can incur physical problems, even with the baby. One couple whom I worked with had many of these problems. The husband abandoned his wife emotionally and beat her during the pregnancy. (I wasn't informed of the beatings until the postpartum visits; otherwise I wouldn't have accepted them as clients.) She gave birth to a healthy 8-pound baby boy, but she hemorrhaged profusely after the placenta was born. After the bleeding was brought under control, she was transported to the hospital where they found no evident cause for her bleeding. Some might say that she needed to get her husband's attention, to scare him so that he would be there for her, or that she caused an emergency to get him to react to show that he loved her. Had I known about the beatings, I would have advised the couple to dismiss any ideas of a homebirth and to go to the hospital. Delivery at home is not acceptable when such disharmony exists.

A couple unwilling to take childbirth education classes—especially a first-time couple—thereby places too much responsibility for the pregnancy and birth on the midwife. In order to have a good homebirth, the couple must take full responsibility for optimally educating themselves. Most communities have ongoing childbirth classes; in communities that do not, the midwife may be able to give them private classes. In my practice, I require that the couple take classes from me or from someone I know. This way I know what they are learning. The couple learns a lot by being around other couples in a class setting, for they learn not only what is being taught, but also that others are experiencing similar feelings. Too often couples feel themselves to be islands, alone with their thoughts and fears. Fears are dispelled through understanding, and understanding can be achieved by educating one's self to the best of one's ability.

Home Birth mentions preexisting chronic diseases such as obesity, diabetes, hypertension, significant cardiac conditions, or emotional disturbances as contraindications for homebirth. Looking at these problems more closely may help you to go over pertinent questions with your birth practitioner.

Obesity

Obesity is a concern during pregnancy. The pregnant woman may not have a healthy diet and may not change her food habits. Her nutritional intake needs to be assessed throughout the pregnancy, so that she can avoid the excessive weight gain that can lead to large babies. A large fetus can transform an easy labor into a problematic labor, involving serious situations such as prolonged labor or shoulder dystocia. With a healthy nutritional intake that is carefully watched and maintained, excessive weight gain can be curbed and a healthy pregnancy can produce a baby of average size. Your doctor or midwife should be consulted.

Diabetes

One of the concerns of diabetes in pregnancy has already been discussed in the material on obesity. Diabetes can bring about a large fetus, producing a more difficult delivery. Diabetes incurs a greater incidence of pre-eclampsia/eclampsia, a higher rate of infection, and a larger volume of amniotic fluid, which in extreme cases may cause cardiorespiratory problems in the mother. Some studies show that the perinatal death rate is higher when the mother has diabetes.

I personally have never worked with a mother who has had diabetes. I have always counseled women with diabetes to consult with a doctor as to whether or not a homebirth is viable for them.

Hypertension

Hypertension is generally termed *high blood pressure*. Although the obstetrical texts list different categories of hypertension that are both common and rare, I will address only the most common problem here. The fear of high blood pressure is that it is indicative of the woman becoming pre-eclamptic, which may turn into eclampsia. By American standards, normal blood pressure is 120/70. It is considered to be getting high when the top number, the systolic, rises as much as 15 to 20 above the normal pressure. The diastolic, the lower number, is also a concern when it starts rising 15 over the average of 70 to 80. Eating properly, lowering one's consumption of alcohol, reducing stress, staying away from foods high in fat content, and getting enough exercise can help maintain a normal blood pressure. A doctor or midwife should be consulted for more information.

Cardiac Conditions

People with conditions that cause discomfort during ordinary physical activity are not appropriate candidates for a birth at home. Such conditions include fatigue, dyspnoea, heart palpitations, and anginal pain. Of special concern are those who have problems with less than ordinary activity or at rest. Since the heart must work harder while in labor, it may be advisable to consult with a doctor if these conditions exists before or during pregnancy.

Emotional Disturbances

As related earlier, the couple's relationship should be harmonious; otherwise, complications can arise during the pregnancy, labor, or delivery. Those having problems should seek professional counseling, and if the problems cannot be resolved, then a hospital may be the safest place for the delivery of the baby.

Grand Multiparity

According to *Home Birth,* no more than five previous births is the criterion for eligibility. Although this is a good guideline, I have known midwives to work with women with more than five previous births. These women were in exceptionally good health. In addition, they ate well, exercised, and had supportive spouses who were willing to take on physical responsibility of the children (giving the mother ample breaks), and were supportive and nurturing during both pregnancy and labor.

Previous Caesarean Section

The old belief "once a caesarean always a caesarean" is a religious dogma that needs to be dispelled. VBAC groups are now debunking this myth. Many proven test cases show that giving birth vaginally after a caesarean is both possible and safe. Cohen and Estner's *Silent Knife* presents exciting facts and statistics on this topic. If this is an issue with anyone, I would strongly recommend reading this book.

Many women who have had previous caesarean sections have given birth at home. A midwife in the county where I live specializes in VBACs at home. With the "rupture" (rather, muscle separation) rate at 2 percent, many parents and professionals believe it is safe to attempt a subsequent vaginal birth at home. Once again, it is important to consult with your midwife or doctor before attempting a homebirth.

Congenital Anomaly

Previous anomalies such as hydrocephaly, spina bifida, cystic fibrosis, and sickle cell anemia need immediate attention upon birth. Consult with your midwife or doctor for more information.

Complications in Previous Pregnancies

As stated in the guidelines, if the woman's pelvic dimensions have proven to cause complications for the birth of a previous normal-size baby, it may be best to keep evaluating the wisdom of a homebirth throughout the pregnancy. Consulting with a midwife or doctor is always advisable in these situations.

In addition to this criterion, I look at the pregnant woman's blood work. I ask the woman if she has had a history of anemia or if she hemorrhaged with any previous births. I ask her to bring me a copy of her CBC (complete blood count) if possible; before I agree to work with her, I will want to look this over. My greatest concern is about anemia. The hematocrit (HCT) and hemoglobin (HGB) are the indicators for this condition; my bottom lines are 36 for HCT and 12 for HGB. The red blood cells carry the oxygen throughout the body. The HCT is the measurement of the percentage of the red blood cells per total blood volume. If the mother is anemic, she and her fetus are not getting enough oxygen. Various complications such as postpartum hemorrhage and fetal distress may arise owing to poor oxygenation of the blood. The mother's cooperation in raising her red blood cell level is essential. Women have told me that they have raised their HCT by eating foods high in iron and by supplementing their diets with herbs and vitamins.

I ask couples to be screened for HIV, as well as any other sexually transmitted disease, toward the end of their pregnancy.

I will not work with any substance abusers, including: alcohol, marijuana, tobacco, or any other drug, be it legal or illegal. Generally, I find that people who want a homebirth are intelligent, well-educated people who care enough about themselves and their babies to stay away from circumstances that may harm them.

Among the woman's reasons for wanting a homebirth should be her goal to be able to labor as she needs to; to avoid the loss of personal control that may be experienced in the hospital; and to have the security of her family and her home during a time when these things are most important and needed.

One of my experiences attending a homebirth illustrates the sometimes complicated attitudes of women toward homebirths. Lynn had heard the beautiful story of her friend's home delivery, and it *was* indeed a wonderful experience. Lynn, who was a very healthy woman, asked me to assist her with the home delivery of her first baby. Her pregnancy was uneventful, so when she went into labor I expected no problems. However, she was very slow to dilate, and her labor progressed very slowly. I found that she was extremely controlled, and when I tried massaging her to get her to relax, she couldn't. She was tight and trying to stay in control instead of relaxing and surrendering her body to let nature do as it is intended. She felt particularily tense in her buttocks and thighs, areas that need to be loose and relaxed in order to get the baby out. After thirty-six hours of strong labor, she had dilated to only 7 centimeters (at 10 centimeters a woman can push the baby out) and was very worn out and tired. Concerned about complications to her and the baby, we both decided she should go to the hospital. Reluctantly, we got things together, climbed into the car, and zoomed off. The contractions became harder in the car and started coming closer together. The hospital was twenty minutes away if we went the speed limit, but it took a lot less time the way we drove that evening. The nurse checked her as soon as she got settled into her private room with curtains and a four-poster bed. Eight centimeters! Lynn seemed more relaxed, even smiling. She chatted with the nurses and seemed right at home. In one sense she was at home, for she worked in a hospital. An hour and a half later, Lynn pushed out a beautiful baby girl who cried very hard, letting us know that she had been through it for a long time, too.

The next day I visited Lynn in her home. With flowers all around and the baby in her arms, she looked like the Madonna herself. "You really wanted to go to the hospital all along, didn't you?" I asked. "I must admit I felt more comfortable once I knew I was going to that hospital." She looked at me sheepishly. "I really wanted to labor at home, but I was too afraid to push the baby out except in the hospital. I was trying to prove something, but my fear got in the way."

About two years later, Lynn gave me a call to say she was pregnant again and wanted a homebirth. She said she realized her previous experience might lead me to turn her down, but she added, "I know that what I want is a birth in my own home. I don't feel such a need to be in control." Eight months later she gave birth to another beautiful baby girl in less than fourteen hours, at home, in her own bed.

With all of these possibilities to take into consideration, the couple's attitude toward life and even death must also be evaluated. A healthy pregnant woman who strives to take optimal care of herself and her unborn child *and* who considers the responsibility of the birth to be hers is a very likely candidate for this very rewarding experience.

Giving birth is an act of nature, an act of God. It has been misplaced in a pathological world by those who fear it and do not trust it. Essentially, it is misunderstood and not respected. Having a baby at home keeps this experience sacred. I feel blessed that my work helps me to experience one of the miracles in nature.

WHAT IS A WATER BIRTH?

Try to remember a day of intense physical or emotional exhaustion. Upon entering a tub or shower of warm water, the tense muscles loosen and your mind relaxes. You feel calmer and perhaps a bit inspired to go on with the work of the day.

Giving birth to a baby takes a lot of hard work. Why not reap the benefits of the relaxing powers of water while doing this hard work? Laboring and giving birth in water has meant a quantum leap in the evolution of childbirth. Not since the late 1960s when the French obstetrician Frederick Leboyer introduced birth with compassion instead of violence has any approach to childbirth so influenced the way a woman can give birth, or the way a baby can receive the first impressions of the world.

A water birth eases the newborn's entry into the world. Both pre- and perinatal psychologists believe that the journey down the birth canal is traumatic for the baby. The fetus in utero is used to hearing his mother's voice and gurgling of her body functions, and to feeling the warmth of the amniotic fluid surrounding him. Then labor begins and something different is happening. The fetus has no comprehension of time, nor is he cognizant that all this forceful squeezing will stop. This process alone may terrify the baby. He then enters a world entirely different from the previous one, with the force of gravity making its first strong impact, with lungs that are not quite ready to function and yet are the only source of his oxygen, and if the umbilical cord is immediately cut, his life line is prematurely severed. The newborn's first impressions can leave an imprint on that person that may last a lifetime. Moving from amniotic fluid to a warm fluid in the birthing tank has a calming effect. It is a familiar, nice resting stop, soothing the baby and protecting him from trauma. The first impressions now suggest to him that this new world is not one of hostility and need not be feared; rather, it can now be seen as a safe, secure, loving environment. Water simply feels good.

Water empowers women, enabling them to labor in a more relaxing and intuitive way. I have assisted many women whom I have found to be too anxious, unable to relax, and therefore unable to collect themselves and tap into their primordial intuition on how to labor. When a laboring mother gets into a tank of warm water, she can relax and find that inner strength that all women share. She can now surrender and let her body tell her how she needs to labor.

She has the freedom to get in and out as she pleases, to move, and to assume whatever position she desires owing to the smaller amount of gravitational pull. Once she is out of the water, gravity has its way. The woman may feel huge, more cumbersome. One mother described to me how laboring in water helped her with her 7- and 8-pound twins. "I could hardly move. I felt like I was floating as opposed to feeling like a beached whale while out of the tank." The buoyancy of water relieves part of that weight. Archimedes found that the weight of water displaced by a body is equal to the weight of that body. With this principle working for the laboring mother, she may feel lighter, seeming to carry the same weight she felt earlier in her pregnancy.

The ideal water temperature for labor is usually between 95 and 100 degrees, whichever feels most comfortable for the mother. The warmth is especially soothing for tired backs and legs, but also comforts the whole body. The warmth of the water is also beneficial for the newborn who comes from a world (the womb's amniotic fluid) where the temperature is approximately 100° F. As it soothes the mother, so it soothes the baby with its fluidity and warmth. Often I have been overjoyed to watch a newborn come out of his mother into the water, open his eyes as if to view his surroundings, and then peacefully shut them. The babies are so at peace—unlike many babies whose births seem to be filled with woe, who emerge with tight-clenched, shuddering fists and grimaced faces filled with terror. There is no comparison.

The vessel that contains the water can fit in even a small room. It can be a hand-built tank, a spa, or a large European bathtub. A few women have labored and given birth in lakes or seas.

Although some mothers use water solely for comfort during labor, many also decide to give birth in the water. Those who are only seeking the relaxing warmth and buoyancy of the water for labor find it so soothing that often they do not want to get out of the water when it is time to push the baby out.

The infant slowly and gently emerges into the water. There is continuity as he enters the safe and familiar environment he knew in the womb: from the amniotic fluid to the water. Many infants appear to be asleep; they don't even know that they are born.

If all goes well, the newborn can remain under the water for a minute or two. Some parents immediately bring the newborn's face out of the water to be in contact with air, while the rest of the body remains in the water for continued relaxation. I like to leave the decision up to the parents when to bring the baby's face to the surface. I have observed that most parents want to bring the face up almost immediately. One couple I worked with was very adamant during their pregnancy that the baby remain under the water for a minute or two, providing, of course, that the baby's condition would permit it. When the baby emerged into the water, the mother was so excited that she immediately scooped the baby up into her arms, holding him close and encouraging him to breast feed. The new mother forgot all about what she had been set on and did what came instinctively, which is what every mother should do.

One couple was not sure whether they wanted to have the baby born in the water. During labor the pregnant mother was using the water for relaxation, and when it came time to push, she found that she didn't want to leave the water. She had a beautiful 10-pound baby boy in the water who peacefully remained under the water for two minutes while the umbilical cord transferred sufficient amounts of oxygen from the placenta. Today this baby boy is a healthy, mischievous fellow with an enormous amount of curiosity. Here was a couple who subscribed to spontaneity with good results. The baby was born so peacefully that he seemed to be asleep. When I tested his reflexes while he was still in the water, his responses were appropriate for a healthy newborn. He was so relaxed after his hard journey. The mother should consult a doctor or midwife on the length of time to leave the baby immersed in the water.

Babies can be and have been born almost anywhere. The questions to ask are, Where does the mother feel most comfortable, and what is safest for both mother and baby? I have known women to travel from Moscow to the Crimean coast of the Black Sea to give birth. They camped in tents while waiting for labor to begin. Some may think this example a bit extreme, but this is where the women felt they wanted to give birth. They did so without complications, and then within hours they began training their babies to swim in the very same sea.

Although water birth is only a little over thirteen years old in the United States, the Russians have been using this method since the

1960s. Approximately three thousand babies have been born in Russia and the Ukraine in this manner.

Using water for relaxation during labor can be beneficial for the baby inasmuch as it calms and soothes the mother. And when the mother feels at ease, so does the baby.

More and more women and men are demanding the use of water to achieve pain relief and to establish a soothing environment for their newborn's entry into the world. Water provides a wondrous alternative to drug use during labor.

3

====

BENEFITS OF WATER BIRTHS FOR MOTHER AND BABY

Water birth has given a whole new definition to birth. Water birth places birth in the context of ecstasy, beauty, fullfillment, empowerment, and strength rather than suffering and disappointment. With water birth childbirth no longer needs to be feared but can be revered, as it was thousands of years ago, before women were made to believe that labor and our monthly bleeding was a curse and a punishment for woman's provocation of sin.

BENEFITS FOR THE MOTHER

Laboring and giving birth in water takes homebirth a step further than its former possibilities because it offers women the chance to move more freely and take up any position she wants and also because it helps her relax, acts as a pain reliever, and reduces energy consumption. These effects contribute to an awareness of her own intuition. Rather than having to succumb to drugs that weaken her both physically and emotionally, with water birth mother and baby attain greater strength to cope with the delivery. As is well known, if the labor is easier on the mother, it will be easier on the baby.

Long before I had heard of giving birth in water, I had witnessed the role of water in childbirth. Over the years I have found that laboring in a warm shower or bath helps the progression of labor. This has been one of the more important tools in my "midwife's bag of tricks." The water has seldom failed to help the mother to relax. I have many fond memories of women standing in the shower with the hot water beating down on their backs, helping them unfold like flower petals to the power of labor. The water was so warm and soothing that many of them did not want to get out when I asked them to. I never gave laboring in water a second thought as to how it worked or why; it just did.

Prior to my experience with water birthing, I shared the conventional phobia about allowing women to labor in a tub with ruptured membranes for fear that both mother and baby would be infected. I never heard of a baby born in water before I became aware of Igor Charkowsky's pioneering water birth work. Now, having attended more than sixty water births, with no such complications, I no longer have that fear about infections. Igor Charkowsky and Michel Odent have reported similar results.

Many people think water is foreign to the birthing process, even though water is such an everyday part of our lives. But fears are natural, and questions of course arise about the baby drowning and about infections. Since our early youth, we have been indoctrinated as to the importance of sterile environments. But are our homes so filled with such terrible bacteria that it is unsafe to give birth in them? If our homes have bad bacteria, what about hospitals? In fact, society consigns people with the worst bacterial infections to hospitals. Hospitals have become acute care centers where those with highly infectious and terminal diseases are in abundance. Mothers are expected to give birth and subject their newborns to this bacteria (which is supposedly contained on certain units and certain floors), whereas most of the "germs" in our homes are with us everyday, forming part of our environment. Perhaps if chickens and pigs were running through our houses, then there might be cause for alarm about germs in the home.

Using the guidelines provided in this book, along with careful screening of the birth practitioner's knowledge and skills—as well as knowing that the most important goal of a labor and delivery is a healthy mother and baby—there are minimal chances for problems, but they can almost certainly be thwarted. Being dogmatic and sticking to an unrealistic idealism about childbirth can only lead to problems and complications. I must reiterate that *the ultimate goal of a labor and delivery is a healthy mother and baby.*

Since my introduction to water births in 1981, I have verified that water is one of the most important vehicles in assisting childbirth. Use of this medium represents one of the main steps in restoring control of birth to where it belongs—to women.

Water's relaxing qualities help to restore this control. A relaxed mind leads to a relaxed body, and vice versa. To be relaxed both physically and emotionally is the key to a quicker and easier labor. To be relaxed is to surrender oneself to one's own body, to open and dilate, allowing the baby to pass through. As soon as the mother begins to relax, she starts surrendering and abandoning her fears, allowing the forces of nature to take over, finding the faith and trust in her body. Having this added strength, she can enter a primitive, meditative state, tapping into her own inherent intuitive powers. The power of water can help this process.

In an article published in *The Lancet* (1983), Dr. Odent wrote of his experiences with women laboring in water.

> We have found, for example, that the mere sight of the water and the sound of it filling the pool are sometimes sufficient stimuli to release inhibitions so that a birth may occur before the pool is full. We have observed that water seems to help many parturients reach a certain state of consciousness where they become indifferent to what is going on around them. . . . During second stage, immersion in warm water seems to help women lose their inhibitions. Most women cry out freely during the last contractions (p. 17).

To lose one's inhibitions while giving birth is much the same thing as losing one's inhibitions while making love. Neither process works when a person is feeling uncomfortable, tight, or restricted. Relying on one's instincts, going into the primitive brain, is tapping into the inherent bodily intuition—to know what to do, to give birth as women have been giving birth for millions of years.

I have seen women fighting labor, trying to control the intensity of the contractions, and unknowingly preventing them from getting stronger. I did this myself when I was in labor with my son Nathaniel. When the contractions seemed to come on like gang-busters, I mentally crossed my legs and tried to control the contractions until my midwife arrived. Waiting for her in my tank of warm water helped me to forget that I was in labor. I was only 3 centimeters dilated, but it seemed hard to adjust to having contractions. The water soothed and caressed me. I felt supported by its buoyancy physically, and it also gave me the feeling of being nurtured, the feeling I had as a child when my mother held me. I became more relaxed, which swept away all the erratic, frantic thoughts pounding in my mind. I remained focused on the thought of the billions of women who had given birth throughout time, a sentiment that also gave me the strength to go on.

Leaving the water felt good, but not for long. With the pull of gravity, I found myself wanting to return to the water's less cumbersome milieu. Back in the water, I got a better grip on the situation. I could move more easily and would get less fatigued. Laboring takes a lot of energy, and I felt better able to conserve my emotional and physical resources when I was able to relax in the warm tank. Once I was able to relax, I could trust that my body knew what to do, and I was able to surrender any control that I mentally had left.

Professionals and mothers alike have experienced this remarkable quality of water. Odent states:

> For one thing, water makes a woman weightless; she can float and no longer has to fight against the weight of her own body during contractions. Furthermore, the warmth of the water reduces adrenaline secretion and relaxes the muscles. Water can also induce alpha brain waves, creating a state of mental relaxation (Odent, 1984, p. 14).

In her evaluation of thirty-one laboring mothers, midwife Myra Smith agrees with Dr. Odent's observations. Smith reported on low-risk women who used warm tub baths during labor. In her abstract, she reports findings of a significant decrease in the anxiety levels of women fifteen minutes after entering the tub. The mean arterial pressure decreased significantly, and pain and distress were also reduced.

During Florence's second water birth, I recall the confirming experience described by both Smith and Odent. Florence labored quite easily with her first water birth and experienced no complications either during or after the birth. I expected the same success for her second delivery, for there were no significant incidences during the pregnancy. When I arrived at the labor, however, I discovered a very uptight Florence. She seemed uneasy and unable to relax. She hadn't been in the water yet and was waiting for the midwives to arrive before entering the tank. I took all her vital signs and found her blood pressure to be very high—around 160/95—whereas it had been absolutely normal throughout her pregnancy. I wasn't too concerned, however, since the protein in her urine was at a normal level. Even so, I mentally resolved to transport her to the hospital if it remained high. I did feel, however, that Florence just needed to relax to bring her blood pressure down.

Florence immersed herself in the water, halfway draped over the wooden frame of the tank. After about fifteen minutes, her mouth changed from a hard, straight line to a sweet, relaxed smile. I waited another fifteen minutes to take the blood pressure. If anything would raise the pressure, it would be stronger contractions, and stronger they were getting. It had been half an hour since the last blood pressure reading. Finally relaxing, Florence looked like a melted doll in the tank. I took her blood pressure and found it had returned to its pregnancy reading of 110/70, absolutely normal! Here was another positive factor of laboring in water. If Florence had been in the hospital, without any water to labor in, she may have had to deal with intervening measures to bring her blood pressure down. Similarly, without water to labor in at the home, if the blood pressure had stayed high, she may have had to be brought to the hospital.

After discussing the labor with Florence, she spoke of how hard it was to deal with the pain. Before she entered the tank, she was in early labor; after she felt the warm waters and began to relax, her contractions came on stronger. Yet she felt she was still able to relax even through the intense "pain."

The "pain" experienced in labor is one of the greatest factors contributing to a woman's inability to relax. It is interesting to me how people of different cultures react to pain. In Western cultures the least bit of discomfort is considered pain. Most people do not accept pain in their lives and have little tolerance for it. In the presence of even the least bit of pain, being accustomed to a comfortable existence, we then reach for a drug to rid ourselves of it as quickly as possible. The thought of dealing with pain for any amount of time represents one of our worst fears. Yes, pain is unpleasant, but are we not losing our courage to deal with even the smallest amounts of pain? Is it possible that we can wipe out pain, both emotional and physical, from day-to-day life? Fear of the "pain" becoming worse is just as significant. Laboring mothers tend to hold back and try to control the pain, wanting it to go away or not to get worse. Many of these women eventually resort to drugs. Through the use of water, the natural hormones can be easily released, putting women in an altered state. Synthetic pain killers are not necessary. They inhibit our own natural hormones, our natural endorphins/opiates. To inhibit the release of these hormones is to intervene, compromising the safety of the mothers and babies in the natural birth process.

Dr. Odent writes:

The fluctuations of hormonal secretions are probably connected with the level of consciousness. One has reason to think that there is an optimum level of consciousness with an optimum secretion of oxytocin and very likely of "endorphins." The role of the system of "endorphins" seems to be obvious when we compare what we observe in the birth room with some scientific data. We observe women who are so different, as if they had drugs, who say they have a strong feeling of well-being between the contractions. These same women say retrospectively that it was as if they had a protection against pain (1981, pp. 45–46).

Dr. Odent writes further:

There are many reasons to think that the system of endorphins is involved during labor and that endogenous opiates can protect both mother and infant against pain. It is also possible to think that this system is still involved at the time of the first contact between the mother and the newborn and participates in the process of "attachment." It is easy to understand that any drug given to the woman in labor can disturb the system of the endorphins (p. 46).

My own hypothesis is that laboring in water affects the oxytocin system. As of yet, no studies have been conducted to confirm this hypothesis.

Serge Wesel, an obstetrician from Belgium, states that a woman's hormonal levels are altered while she is laboring in water:

> Studies have already shown that cortisol, beta endorphin, and prolactin levels are significantly changed in women laboring in water. The secretion of endorphins, cortisol, and prolactin, B-endorphin and cortison was higher in air [out of the birthing tank] as opposed to water, while prolactin was higher in the group laboring in the bath.

Through my work with women laboring in water as well as in the traditional home birth setting, it is inevitable when a woman starts relaxing in labor her hormones will kick in and she will start progressing faster and with more rhythm. The labor becomes more efficient, enabling the laboring mother to use the tools that she learned in her childbirth class and those that are inherent to her.

The Family Center Associates, Inc. of Albuquerque, New Mexico, incorporates tub-bathing into the labor process. They have found that warm water (98 to 101° F) provides pain relief and augments the progress of labor. The midwives associated with the group wrote of the easy dilations of the women laboring in water and reported that the new mothers' temperatures remained normal for three days after delivery. No infections were found.

Many factors influence the perception of pain. Everyone has a different pain threshold, with some of us able to tolerate more than others. For the majority of women labor is intense; plainly, it hurts. A new mother cannot know what to expect of labor. If she goes into labor unprepared, fear can overwhelm her, wiping out any intuitive responses that she may be called upon to make. If she has prepared herself properly, has good emotional support, and has retained her confidence in her womanhood, she will perceive pain in a different manner—that is, as a miraculous sensation that only a woman's body can accomplish, which happens only a few times in one's life. A mother who has given birth before may be aware of the possibilities to come and may be able to deal with the contractions better on an intellectual level. Even so, a certain percentage of pain exists.

In the childbirth world some schools of thought maintain that the word *pain* has negative connotations. It is true that the intensity of the contractions needs to be viewed in a more positive light. The pain of labor is different from most of the other pain we may experience in our lifetimes. Unlike all other pains, the pain of labor has a productive outcome. As the mother is laboring, she is witnessing one of the great miracles of life. Her body is working, actually giving birth to life. The outcome of this pain is usually positive—a beautiful baby.

In some circumstances, the nonreferral to pain is carried a bit too far. Parents may develop a head-in-the-sand attitude and deny any possibility of pain. This is just as negative an approach as having too much fear of pain, especially with new parents who haven't experienced labor. When laboring mothers are not psychologically prepared, the pain can be overwhelming. Recognizing that there are no guarantees in nature is also a matter of trusting in one's body. The laboring mother does have to deal with the reality that nature can, at times, be unpredictable as well as uncomfortable.

Women who have labored or given birth in water cannot imagine going through the birthing process without water. From a midwife's perspective, I feel sad for those women whom I see laboring without the soothing effects of warm water.

BENEFITS FOR THE BABY

She was born under water. When she emerged, it was with open and exploring eyes. Not the passive arrival haze through which an "alert" demeanor is considered optimum, but *beyond* newborn alert to "conscious." Like the difference from having "reflexes" to initiating movement—being self-motivated. Halley made swimming motions and felt her mama's heartbeat from the outside in the fluid water world which was her first earthside matrix. She appeared to have been born without any trauma, but in trust fulfilled; the way conscious beings in this century-of-the-child have hoped. . . . Halley is a harbinger of the new species— people who arrive here untraumatized, united with the original love which called them forth. Fully conscious, connected to their feelings without drug stupor, retreat from primal pains or maternal/paternal separation (Jeanine Parvati Baker, midwife/mother).

Similar accounts are given by the numerous other ecstatic mothers who have given birth to their babies in water. From a midwife's perspective, I was attracted to water births not only for the laboring mother, but also for the newborn.

Several psychologists believe that the labor and delivery process may have a lasting influence on the fetus. Groups such as the International Society of Pre- and Perinatal Psychology and Medicine are studying a number of theories positing that newborns are affected by their births. One psychologist, Thomas Verney, author of *The Secret Life of the Unborn Child* (1981), has worked with several patients who were able to recall their feelings at the time of their births. Several of these patients had deep psychological scars that were traceable to forceps or caesarean deliveries or to a rough delivery; most of the time their scars involved the alienation of mother and newborn. Recurring nightmares, fears, anxieties, and even headaches have been attributed to birth trauma. Through hypnosis, breathing techniques, psychoanalysis, and other means, these traumas have been brought to the surface and hopefully treated successfully.

David Chamberlin, in his book *Babies Remember Birth* (1988), gives several accounts of people remembering their births. He states that young children, upon first learning to speak, will sometimes verbalize incidents from their births. They may question certain things such as the bright lights in the room or express feelings painful to them. Others may describe coming down chutes or being in a swimming pool. Dr. Chamberlin also presents stories of children relating their births, which match the stories of their parents or birth attendants.

The understanding that newborns have feelings has only recently been acknowledged by the greater medical community. Leboyer's book, *Birth Without Violence* (1975), turned the heads of both parents and professionals. Leboyer's theory that perhaps newborns are conscious and feel at birth challenged and questioned the written-in-stone act of holding the baby upside down and slapping the infant on the behind. Leboyer also questioned using the bright hospital lights that are so blinding to the newborn. Along with the segregation from the mother came the cold rooms which are much too frigid for the newborn's inner thermometer, which hasn't yet learned to reach a balance. Perhaps Leboyer is most famous for returning the baby to a medium that she is most familiar with, a medium that she has spent nine months in. Leboyer observed that putting the baby into a small tub of warm water soothes and relaxes the baby. Once in the tub, babies crying are becalmed. In his book, Leboyer asks some very simple but profound questions. The answers are obvious but until recently have been long ignored. He points out that babies cry at birth, as if in terror, and he questions whether this is not a sign of pain or anguish. Do we as adults and children, he asks, not have these responses when we encounter similar situations? He also asks why we assume that birth is less painful for the child than for the mother; why we assume that this "thing" cannot feel, hear, or see; why we treat "it" as such an object.

My own question is, when does this "thing" become a person? When he starts rolling over? Walking? Talking? The newborn is not born equipped with the gift of speech. The newborn's communication is different; he or she speaks not with words but through crying. Leboyer asks what more proof do we need of the newborn's distress when we hear the howling, see the white-knuckled fists, and the grimacing, terror-stricken faces? Is this the way a baby needs to look and feel at birth? How many times has a newborn been described as ugly? In all my years of practice as a midwife, I have never seen an ugly newborn. And never have I seen a terror-stricken face on a child who has just entered the world through water. If the fetus is as cognizant in the last month as many believe, the disturbance of his tranquility could be quite alarming.

Imagine yourself peacefully reclining in the bath. A candle is flickering, producing the only light in your comfortable little world. Suddenly the plug is pulled. With your head down you are sucked through the narrow tight pipes, the walls squeezing and grinding against you, slowly packing you downward. Your head is compressed so hard that the plates in your skull begin to shift to fit into the narrow passageway of the drain pipe. You think to yourself, "what is going on?" "How long can this last?" "Will it ever stop?"

Then it does stop after your head gets squeezed even tighter and protrudes out of the hole of the drain pipe, with a tight rope wrapped around your neck. As you come from the absolute dark, somebody then turns on the bright beams of their car lights directly into your eyes and hangs you by your feet from a tree limb. As if all this isn't enough, a giant paddle is solidly smacked on your bare behind. You are then taken away and put in a room with half a dozen screaming people lying around you. Imagine this being your first introduction to a foreign country, or for that matter another planet.

Why do people believe that newborns feel nothing? They do feel. That's all, in fact, they can do. They feel every little sound, every little movement, every little sensation. They hear their mother's voice, they feel her belly bump a door knob, they listen to her digestion, and when she bathes in the sun, they see the filtered light of the sun's rays.

We treat the body of the newborn delicately. "Be careful with her head." "Place the baby gently in the crib." However, we fail to acknowledge all the other aspects of this being, especially at birth. Why should the newborn have to arrive in a world that is so totally different from the one he is used to? Why is it inconceivable to so many that a gentle, nonviolent entry into this world can be easily obtained, a place where similar sensations are rendered to make the newborn's entry a loving environment. Not only can this kind of entry be easily obtained, but also it is necessary for the child's psychological development. Igor Charkowsky believes that children born under water are less prone to sickness and are very strong spiritually.

Leboyer speaks of newborns perceiving sounds as fish in water, "modulated and transformed." These sounds are muted inside the waters of the womb. Upon arrival, the newborn is blasted with sounds—cries of "it's a boy!" or the screams of the mother while she pushes the baby out. Being born into the water mutes these sounds, just as they are muted inside the womb. The vulnerable ears are protected by the silence of the waters.

Leboyer also reminds us of the sensitivity of the skin. "Its skin—thin, fine, almost without a protective surface layer—is as exposed and raw as tissue that has suffered a burn. The slightest touch makes it quiver" (1975, p. 19). In my midwifery practice, my partner and I always made a point of picking the softest blanket we could find to wrap the baby in. We wouldn't pin the diapers onto the newborn, but gently tucked them underneath, just in case the newborn decided to move her bowels. I always love touching a newborn's skin. It is as soft as velvet, pink, smooth, and translucent. The skin is the greatest receptor, the largest organ of our bodies. It, too, is fresh, new, and untouched by the outside world. The receptors are wide open and sensitive to any abrasiveness and change in temperature. At birth the young are unable to regulate their own body temperature, and so they are bundled up in warm clothing immediately after birth. If they are lucky, someone has turned up the heat in the room.

Abner Levkoff writes of "the functional integrity of the tissues [of the newborn] with the highest metabolic rate, like the central nervous system, tolerate the least change in temperature. . . . the oxygen consumption of the fetus at term compares with that of the resting adult in a neutral thermal environment (1982, p. 104). He also states that an increase in heat production is needed and that preserving heat loss is essential for keeping the newborn's metabolism functioning well. Since, as he points out, the newborn has a body mass of 5 percent and a body surface area of 15 percent of that of the adult, the newborn is especially susceptible to heat loss.

The water in the tank aids the thermal regulation and adaptations of the newborn, for it is the same temperature as the amniotic fluid. Battling with the new elements is not necessary; adaption to life outside the womb can be slow and easy.

When the child is born in water, the skin is caressed by the silky fluidity, recreating a sensation that has been experienced for the first nine months of life. Water is soothing to the skin after the long, arduous journey down the birth canal. The skin may now be bruised or even cut. The warmth is soothing, reminiscent of the warm fluidity of the womb, bringing back a feeling of familiarity, safety, and security. The water doesn't sting or burn the skin as the air is thought to; it is simply nurturing for this new person who has gone through such a long, difficult journey.

The lungs are just as sensitive as the skin. Leboyer theorizes the infant's difficulty of adjusting to having air in the lungs. He compares this adjustment to that of a first-time smoker when he goes through the violent reactions of having the foreign intrusion into his lungs.

The air not only is intruding, but it is also intruding prematurely. Cutting the umbilical cord before the cord stops pulsating prevents sufficient amounts of blood from entering the baby. The blood is the oxygen carrier that has been the growing fetus's lifeline for nine months. The baby's lungs are not quite ready to be on their own; a physiological process still needs to occur. The alveoli, which are the little sacs in the lungs that perform the oxygen/carbon dioxide exchange, are not immediately ready to start functioning. It takes only a short amount of time, but the alveoli have not yet popped open to do their chemical exchange. If the umbilical cord is cut prematurely, the newborn may go into respiratory distress if the lungs are not ready to start functioning. This distress is not necessary, as the placenta is still pumping blood (and oxygen) to the newborn for minutes after the birth. Touching the umbilical cord, one can feel the strong pulsating, the flowing of the blood through the arteries and veins, nourishing the newborn with blood and oxygen. According to Leboyer:

> If the cord is severed as soon as the baby is born, this puts the brain into a state of oxygen deprivation. The baby's entire system reacts as if an alarm has gone off. Respiration is thrown into high gear as a response to aggression. The baby's body and voice appear to be in a state of panic; the limbs move in a frenzied state, the cry is that of someone who is being terrorized (1975, p. 46).

Abner Levkoff states: "The alveoli are distended with a volume of lung fluid which approximates 30 ml/kg of body weight. This fluid volume is equal to the functional residual volume of air that will take its place when breathing begins, and the pulmonary fluid is almost completely absorbed 15 minutes after birth by pulmonary lymphatics and capillaries" (1982, p. 105). This is nearly the same amount of time that the placenta, which pumps the blood to the newborn, needs to separate itself from the wall of the uterus.

Being born into water provides a place of transition for the newborn where he or she can adjust to life in this new dimension. The physiological adaptations to extrauterine life can proceed at the newborn's own pace. If all is going well, the parents and the birth attendant may elect to leave the baby under the water for a minute or two. The water keeps the umbilical cord moist and warm, which slows down the hardening of Wharton's jelly (the protective jelly surrounding the arteries and vein in the umbilical cord) and prevents premature pressure on these blood vessels. Therefore, the baby is allowed to continue getting nourishment through the umbilical cord, thus giving the lungs the time they need. The life-rhythms of the newborn need to be respected. Charkowsky believes that to be born in water gives the child "an extra good start in life." He believes that the newborn is exposed to gravity too suddenly after the weightlessness that is experienced in the womb. Charkowsky also believes that the lesser force of gravity on the newborn's brain reduces the necessity for oxygen by 60 to 70 percent. He, too, is concerned about the sudden impact of oxygen on the lungs. He feels that the gravity and the premature imposition of oxygen on the lungs affects the very sensitive brain functions.

The fetus's last few months in utero become restrictive, giving her less room to move. The big ocean has now become a little pond holding the baby uncomfortably tight. Curling up, with her head tucked tightly in, she tries to make as much room as possible. Labor begins and the tightness increases, pushing against her head and spinal column, twisting it as if she were a contortionist. When emerging into the water, the infant may experience a greater feeling of freedom, of serenity such as Leboyer describes as the "Golden Age" in the uterus, when the fetus is small enough to have a floating sensation. The spine is also supported. When the newborn's face is brought to the surface, the baby can float, uncurling the spine. Because only the back and sides of the baby's head are supported by the water, the baby can experience freedom of movement owing to the water's lesser amount of gravity. The spine is less stressed than it would be if the baby were lying on a firm or a hard surface. What a stark contrast this experience is to the one lived by the baby who is held upside down and whose spine is snapped straight.

Newborns in water commonly make swimming motions as they did in the womb. They appear peaceful and at rest, and they have a contented glow on their faces. They become weightless, almost free of their bodies, floating as they once did in the earlier days of their development. Their arms move about as graceful ballerinas, while their feet thrust about like olympic swimming champs, as if they have been doing this all their lives. And well they have, for these little sea creatures leaving their mother's womb are returning to a place of no restrictions, happy and contented. When they leave the water, they cry; put them back into the tank, and they are happy again.

In the hospital setting, newborns are often left alone. The new mother may have just had surgery, and the drugs have not worn off yet. Perhaps the delivery was difficult for her, and she wants some time to recover and to rest. The newborn is then taken to the nursery and left with the nurse or just put in the crib. For the past nine months the fetus has never been away from his mother. Now he retreats inside himself, feeling abandoned after the torture he has just endured. Now, like a prisoner, he must endure the isolation that others see fit to impose on him.

Instead, he could be floating in the familiar warm water with his mother and father with him. Perhaps a brother or sister is there touching his skin, remarking how soft he is. The new mother has had to expend far less energy during the birth due to laboring in the water. She is awake and alert, able to be there for him. No drugs have been needed. The newborn doesn't have to retreat within himself; there is no reason to. He feels safe and opens up like a flower, welcoming the world, viewing life in a positive manner.

Perhaps we should now rewrite birth, making it a time when coming into the world is a soothing, gentle experience for the newborn. It should mark an entry that shows life is not cruel, but a place where one is welcomed and loved. In his book Leboyer stresses that we need to speak the baby's own language, an unspoken language that has to do with touch. The water's touch, with its gentle familiarity, tells the baby that it is okay to be here. The water speaks in a loving manner, a language that the newborn remembers. Their alarm systems do not have to go off; they do not have to feel they are under attack. These water babies don't have to be calmed, for most of them are asleep when they enter the water. Theirs is a slow and gentle transition from one life to another, ensuring bonding.

Why is bonding so important? Bonding is simply that old-fashioned feeling of falling in love that brings mother and baby closer together. Bonding is important not only for mother and child, but also for the father and siblings of the newborn. Many believe it strengthens the family ties, lowers the possibility of child abuse, and lessens the jealousy of the older children. Bonding also helps establish breastfeeding; exploring the baby, holding, and touching produce closer feelings.

Water assists with the bonding in so many ways. Some may cringe, seeing the baby come into the world with blood all over him, and may call him "dirty." With a water birth the baby is washed clean at birth in the very first environment into which he is born.

Because the first instant of birth is the very first introduction to life, we owe this period a tremendous amount of respect. Just as we want to make a good first impression on someone new whom we meet, so too do we want to make a loving impression of life on the newborn. This is a very fragile time. Some believe that first impressions count, actually setting the very foundations of what life is about. We live in a society where everything is hurried and time is pressed. Must life start out this way? In our first moments, should we be rushed into life, into meeting schedules?

Most of us think that it is normal or healthy to hear the baby wail at birth. Upon witnessing the tranquility of a water birth, some react in a troubled manner, concerned that the baby needs to be clearing his lungs. Although educated about water births, some parents and professionals are not prepared for the peacefulness of the newborn. When we assume that the grimaced faces of newborns are normal, essentially, we are saying that it is normal to suffer at birth. But birth and suffering need not be one and the same. Water birth can provide the baby a smooth transition into life.

Life affects who we are and how we react to things. Therefore, coming into the world in a gentle manner as our first introduction to life can only imprint gentleness and a feeling of security and being loved on us. What happens later on may disturb some of this tranquility, but the basic foundation is there for the water babies to grow on and to forge on through the world without fear.

4

===

PRENATAL CARE AND PREPARATION

The importance of prenatal care cannot be overemphasized. It is one of the essential factors that contributes to a beautiful birth, that is, a healthy mother and baby. Without good prenatal care, complications that may occur in pregnancy are overlooked, threatening the well-being of both mother and baby, evolving into problems and complications during labor and delivery.

Few of us know exactly what good prenatal care is. We rush into the doctor or midwife's office, race through a prenatal exam, and leave in five to seven minutes. Often the practitioner has little time for questions and answers, and has little information on nutrition. We can be left in the dark, with worries that chip away at our emotional well-being. Prenatal care can and should cover much more of the whole person than what is covered in the contemporary medical world.

We live in an era when responsibility for one's own basic health care is being handed over to those who sit in the seats of authority. Yes, we do need people to guide us and help us to make the proper decisions concerning our health. Yet many people are questioning the manner in which our health care is being delivered. We need to educate ourselves so that we can make intelligent decisions and not just blindly hand the responsibility for our health over to someone else. This sets the practitioner on a high pedestal, giving that person all the power. When something goes wrong, the practitioner is blamed; then come the lawsuits.

For approximately the last sixty years, women have become accustomed to handing over their birthing power to the godlike image of the doctor. Instead of being empowered, she is raped of the inherent, instinctive bodily process of giving birth. Many women today automatically hand over their rights to doctors without any question. It is as if they are saying, "Take me. I am not qualified to give birth without modern technology." Many know no other way.

Selecting a midwife or a doctor is the next important step if you have decided to have an underwater birth. Throughout my practice as a midwife, I have found that one of the most important aspects as a caregiver is to establish a mutual loving rapport with the mother and father. It is important to establish a bond, to know how the couple's emotional relationship is doing, and to establish an open means of communication. I also like to be available to answer questions and give support. When the pregnant couple and I are choosing whether or not to work together, I let them know that I am not attending the birth in a position of control. The birth attendant serves as an adviser and an emergency backup.

Another important role of the midwife is to help the couple decide if a water birth is really what they want. Sometimes a homebirth and water birth can be romanticized; couples may think that because their neighbor had a wonderful time with a water birth, the pregnant couple will too. The possibilities of a good outcome are very high, but still the couple needs to examine what their motivations and incentives are for electing this particular method of birthing.

A couple once came to me requesting a water birth. One of the first questions that I ask every couple is, "What made you decide to have a water birth?" The pregnant mother piped in, "Well, Henry's former wife had a water birth, and he wants me to have one too. I don't want to feel any pain, so I would like to labor in the water." On talking further to the woman, she raised an eyebrow and said, "You do carry pain killers if the water doesn't take away the pain, don't you?" All the sirens and the red flags went up in my mind. This woman obviously belonged in the hospital. First, she was asking for a water birth merely to please her husband, not for herself. Second, she didn't want to deal with any pain. I expressed my concern to the couple and asked them to seriously question their motives for having a water birth. A few months later, they wrote me, thanking me and informing me that they had decided that a hospital birth was best for them. The woman was actually terrified to stay at home and experience the pain.

Screening is extremely important in making sure that the practitioner and the couple can have a good relationship. Pregnancy and delivery is one of the most important times in a woman's as well as the baby's life, and so it should be treated as a spiritual experience. The birth attendant should respect this time, as well as the needs and wishes of the mother, father, and baby. The birth attendant should be there not only to guide the mother, but also to empower her to use her intuition to be healthy during her pregnancy and when giving birth. The midwife brings many special skills with her during these nine months. Among them are guidance and the ability to use emergency techniques if needed. These skills are essential and must not be underrated. Both the practitioner and the birthing couple should leave ego satisfaction and the need for power and control behind. Any good birth attendant receives her rewards from a healthy delivery, as well as from helping the couple achieve their desired way of birth as safely as possible during the pregnancy and the parturition (providing, of course, that it is within the mother and baby's best interests healthwise).

The midwife or doctor should be asked specific questions pertaining to water births. I have heard of problems occurring when midwives or doctors are assisting a water birth simply because of consumer demand by the parents, not because they believe in it or understand its value. It is important to believe in this process, just as it is important to believe in the natural process of birth. I thoroughly agree that a practitioner should respond to a couple's wishes. However, if the attendant is not well educated about water births, fear may be present at the birth, unnecessary interventions could be used, and complications could arise, which would then be incorrectly attributed to the water birth. Believing that water is helpful during labor and is beneficial for both mother and baby is a pretty sound reason for a practitioner to attend a water birth.

In my practice I have seen no complications that I sincerely felt were due to the mother giving birth in the water. Complications have arisen, but they would have anyway whether the birth was in or out of water. If the doctor or midwife feels comfortable with the situations at the birth, a more relaxed atmosphere will enable everyone present to relax—most importantly, the laboring mother.

If the midwife or doctor is new to water birthing, he or she should be asked to do some research to enable the mother to feel comfortable with the birthing process, so that she will be able to make educated decisions during the pregnancy and labor. A lot of information on the subject is readily available in the medical literature, midwifery journals, and childbirth magazines.

Speaking to other practitioners who have attended water births is also very helpful for the midwife, for professional questions can be answered and may ease the fears of anyone taking on legal and medical responsibility for the birth. I found it very confirming to speak with couples who had gone through the water birth process. In the early 1980s these people were hard to find, but I persisted, wanting to know precisely what kind of people were having these births, what the outcomes were, and whether they were satisfied. All these couples were well-educated people with their feet firmly planted on the ground. Their enthusiasm for birthing in water was very contagious, and the mothers' descriptions of their gentle labors and deliveries were reassuring.

The midwife may sometimes be fortunate enough to attend a water birth as an observer. Water births are now more popular and so are more easily accessible for those who need this learning experience. Some mothers are glad to share their birth experience, while others consider their labor to be a private and intimate matter. The information gained from attending a water birth can be handed from midwife to midwife when it is first-hand experience. This, in fact, is the way the knowledge of midwifery has been handed down since the beginning of time.

Videos of water births are available. These can be reassuring and ease the viewer's mind that this is truly a wonderful way to have a baby. Karil Daniels of Point of View Productions located at 2477 Folsom St., San Francisco, Calif. 94110, phone (415) 821-0435, has produced a tape depicting an underwater birth in the United States as well as the work of Igor Charkowsky in Russia and Michel Odent in France. Daniels has also issued a resource book on underwater births.

I have found it very important for anyone who attends a water birth to be well educated about the subject, so that they do not bring their fears and anxieties to the birth. There is nothing worse than having a birth attendant present who is vexing every moment of the labor.

PSYCHOLOGICAL PREPARATIONS

A positive attitude is one of the most important ingredients for a healthy pregnancy and delivery, whereas fear is the greatest contributor to complications during labor. Basically, it is fear of the unknown and the fear that women have been fed about childbirth from their earliest years. In the American culture and many Western cultures generally, society has led us to believe that we must "suffer" while giving birth. The Hollywood movies depict hysterical women screaming in the background, while the men are far removed, pacing outside, smoking their cigars. Even the Bible condemns women to suffering during childbirth, as depicted in Genesis 3:8, 16–17: "The Lord God said to the woman, 'I will greatly increase your pains in childbearing; with pain you will give birth to children." It is no wonder women are so afraid of their own bodies. For the last sixty years, women have been isolated from each other during childbirth. Before this time family members and neighbors would routinely be present to help at the birth. Women were able to see each other give birth and to see that birth was a common, everyday, *natural* occurrence. No mysteries were attached to the event. Women knew what to expect, and so their fears were dispelled.

Being in touch with one's own fears is very important. It may be a fear that is very simple in origin, and once looked at and questioned, it may appear to be quite silly. Take some time to sit quietly, to gather your thoughts, to meditate. Focus on what you are afraid of, and formulate your fears into questions so that research may be done to answer these questions, thus alleviating the fears—perhaps by reading books on the topic or by finding somebody who has a lot of experience with the topic of concern. Taking a childbirth education class is one of the best ways to obtain information. I have found that reading as many books about pregnancy and childbirth as possible will assure women that their bodies will know what to do while in labor. Should complications arise, being educated about the complications one may face and the different ways of handling them is very empowering, allowing women to participate in the decisions that may have to be made. Being informed, knowing what they are dealing with, helps women to feel they are in control of their bodies and can help them find the strength not to surrender that control to someone else.

A healthy attitude in parents starts even before conception. Preparing physically and spiritually to conceive, to carry a new life, takes some thought and readjustment. Basically, it changes one's idea of what is important. I recommend Jeanine Parvati Baker's book *Conscious Conception* (1986), which is a good resource on this topic. Making a good start at the beginning is a great way to get on a positive track.

Taking time out and quieting one's self every day for even a few minutes is always important, but especially when pregnant. In examining one's self, ask what is important for you that you want to have happen during the pregnancy. What would you like to change in your life during the pregnancy? What would the ideal birth be for you? Ideally, it is important to make pregnancy and labor a time of fulfillment. And when this is not possible, it is important to recognize what good has come out of the experience, what changes could have been made, and to be happy that mother and baby are healthy.

Most women undergo some psychological changes and experience feelings of inadequacy while pregnant. Facing these changes and discussing them with the midwife will help encourage a better relationship and will allow the midwife to become familiar with the pregnant mother's needs and with her personality.

Feelings of inadequacy are often due to social conditioning. Some women are afraid of losing their figures and of not appearing sexy to their husbands. Yet many men find pregnant women very sexy and get turned on seeing a pregnant woman.

A pregnant woman should be proud of her big belly. Flaunt it! She should be happy she is with child. Being pregnant is a beautiful state both physically and spiritually. Watching the different stages of pregnancy, month after month, is a unique and holy experience. The woman's body changes so rapidly during these months that to follow the stages constitutes a course in anatomy and physiology in itself. It is truly fascinating how the woman's body will slowly go back to its former shape after the baby is born, especially if the baby is breastfeeding.

Pregnant women also express concern about losing their independence. Some women may be working and are anxious that they may become dependent on their husbands. Women having their first baby are especially fearful of the change a baby will make in their lives. Some even fear the dependency that the baby will have on them and the full responsibility the child will impose on them, particularly if little or no help is expected from the father. The insecurities can come in many guises, and every pregnant mother has at least one. The key to solving these problems is for them to get in touch with exactly who they are, to ask questions, and to educate themselves about midwifery, obstetrics, pregnancy, and birth.

During pregnancy communication is one of the most important tools for alleviating these problems. Communication is important not only for the father and mother, but also for their birth attendant. Sitting down together and calmly discussing problems may not always clear the air immediately, but it may open the channels for more communication. It is very important for prospective parents to discuss their concerns, problems, and issues during the pregnancy, and to resolve as many questions as possible. Problems may arise in labor due to suppressed feelings. For example, a woman who tends to keep her problems to herself and to suppress them during the pregnancy may find it difficult to let go and relax during labor; her cervix may be unable to open and dilate, just as she was unable to open to her self and her partner during the pregnancy. It is important to be able to get in contact with one's own feelings and to verbalize them. Enjoying the pregnancy is so important for the mother, which ultimately affects the unborn baby. A mediator such as the midwife or a counselor can help with problems that cannot be resolved between the parents. Or perhaps some separate work can be accomplished with a midwife or a psychologist.

The father may be going through his own fears and insecurities. Many men keenly feel the weight of responsibility that a new person imposes on them. They may already be struggling financially and may be wondering how they will be able to make ends meet, especially when the wife may have to stop working. Somehow these problems resolve themselves.

A common complaint of pregnancy from the woman's viewpoint is her feeling that she is not getting enough attention from her husband. She wants to be with him more, and craves his attention and affection. He, on the other hand, feels that he is being the dutiful husband simply by bringing in more money and being a good provider. This seems to be the perennial battle of the sexes, pregnant or not. Remember that there are always two sides to the story. Communication and making compromises can help in these situations.

Getting in Touch with One's Womanliness

Womanliness means something different to every woman. Most women agree that it is important to do some soul searching as to the precise meaning of this term to the individual, especially during pregnancy. A woman may want to work on such things as intuition, empowering herself, obtaining her own inner strength, and examining what is important for her heart and soul. I have found that this means sorting out one's beliefs as to what is right and wrong. We all have a conscience, which reminds us what is right and wrong.

Many women may have already penetrated to these areas of their being, but there is always room for fine tuning. In the 1960s, the feminist revolution produced an intense search for more self-awareness by women, and women began seeking an identity separate from men. Since then, many women's groups have been formed to help empower women in many different aspects of life that were either closed to them before or have now been reintroduced.

In this new age of the career woman, women are still struggling for equality and equal pay. Precisely because of career considerations, some women postpone pregnancy and mothering. Women undergo quite an adjustment of lifestyle when, after a hard day's work, instead of putting their feet up and reading the newspaper, they have to switch gears, becoming housewife and mother. This change frequently produces conflict in the home and a reevaluation of family roles. In this situation, many women complain that they don't have the time for self-awareness, especially if they are single mothers. Thus, making time for quiet moments or interests beyond work and family is easier said than done, especially during pregnancy. However, the pregnant woman does need time to replenish her strength. This may mean just sitting quietly, meditating, joining women's support groups, or getting together with some good friends.

A lioness is in every woman, especially during pregnancy and motherhood, although for some of us other role models and societal expectations have squelched this instinct. This inner strength is potentially in every woman, however, and it needs to be built on throughout pregnancy. The pregnant woman needs to feel so strong about herself and her body that, if need be, she could give birth completely alone without mate, midwife, or doctor, for essentially, giving birth is a solitary activity. Only the laboring mother can give birth; no one can do it for her. People may be able to give advice, comfort, and some assistance, but it is the mother's body and spirit that is giving birth. If she doesn't feel self-assured, then problems may arise. Here I do not mean to encourage women to give birth alone, which would be a dangerous situation at best. The point I am making is that women need to be in a state of mind where they are dependent, emotionally and spiritually, only on themselves and their God.

So find out what your womanhood means to you. It may have to do with your beliefs, your way of life. You may be a feminist, an outdoors woman, an intellectual, a career woman, an earth mother, a housewife and mother, or a worshiper of the Goddess. Or you may be a combination of all these. The point is to find out what feels to be your truth and what feels right for you.

One tool that will help determine this truth is that age-old womanly intuition; it could also be called "common sense." In these modern times women seem to be straying farther and farther from using their intuition. For many, intellectual rationalizing has taken the place of the intuitive tool that is our birthright. Intuition is being able to find that place in one's soul where one knows right from wrong and one's truth. When playing with young children, I am always impressed with their intuitive knowledge. Many are able to make clear decisions, knowing what is right for them. We need to know how to call upon that intuition. One mother described it as a feeling deep in her "guts," or a "gut-level" feeling. I believe we have all had these feelings at one time or another. The more we use it and trust in it, the easier and quicker we will be able to find our intuition. It is woman's unique sixth sense.

Remembering to use our intuition instead of our intellectual aspect can, when appropriate, be the first step to empowerment. Women's groups encourage women to develop and use this sense. Discussions with women about how to procure this sixth sense have produced various ideas on what intuition is and how to enhance it. Given that everyone has the ability to use their intuition, here are some ideas that will help strengthen this ability.

Being Alone in Nature

We are creatures of nature just as is the deer or the fox. Our natural surroundings, however, have decidedly become unnatural; steel and glass and a fast-paced life propel us at high velocities through time and space. Living in the woods is foreign to the great majority of us these days; for most of us, the city park is the closest we ever come to the natural habitat of our ancestors. The hustle-bustle of everyday life makes it difficult to take time to relax and enjoy life. Ideally, we should all live on a wooded acre with a stream running through the property, but, barring that, every woman should take time out to do things in nature that will help her relax, thus allowing the natural instincts of childbirth to surface.

Going camping is one way for us all to slow down: to listen to the rhythms of our surroundings; to take joy in the simple everyday scenes of nature like butterflies flitting from flower to flower, the squirrel scampering up the tree with a big nut in its mouth, the deer grazing gracefully in a meadow; to sit in deep quiet, feeling our own body rhythms, slowing down enough to get to know our self apart from all the foreign input that a day brings. These things quiet us, not only in our mind but also in our soul. Living in Sonoma County, California, which borders the Pacific, enables me to go to the ocean. It is there I go to clear my head, to get answers to difficult questions. Some say the negative ions around bodies of water soothe and relax us. The sound of the ocean, the beauty of the rugged rocks and cliffs, remind me that I am part of this ecosystem, as were my ancestors who swam and fished on similar beaches. I am a link in a chain that goes back to when women would simply squat where they were to have their babies.

I often suggest that pregnant women go to nature to relieve their stress. Women who want to have a water birth find sitting by a stream or a pond to be just as gratifying as going to the ocean. They speak of their affinity with water, how it gives them an inner strength that lies deep within their souls and makes them feel they can accomplish anything by themselves, especially birth. The woman is the only person who can orchestrate the labor and give birth to the baby. Women need to know that they are strong, emotionally and spirtually, and that their bodies can perform all that is necessary to labor and give birth. This is where the intuition comes in. Intuition is the most important tool that a women can have when giving birth. It is her inner voice; it tells her what is best for her while laboring. It is not a voice of fear telling her she can't stand the "pain" and needs drugs. It is knowing when to walk around the yard to get the baby down lower into the pelvis, knowing when to lie on her side or when to squat. Recognizing her intuition enables a woman to hold on to her power, her inherent laboring rights, and not relinquish them to a doctor or a midwife, allowing them to decide what to do. She is going through the labor, she feels what is happening to her body and knows what is needed. With faith in herself, and support from her close ones, she will learn to trust her intuition. Intuition feels right. If something feels wrong or amiss, the woman should listen. Her intuition is telling her something. Women should be careful not to confuse their intuition with preconceived mindsets. It is easily done when a woman wants things to go a certain way. For example, during her pregnancy a woman may have dreamed of having certain things happen, but labor may not progress the way she envisioned it. Trying to make things happen the way she wants them to defeats her intuition and takes the control of labor and delivery away from her body and invests it in her preconceptions. It is important that each woman learns to differentiate between intuition and dogmatic stubborness.

Another simple way I found to empower myself during pregnancy was gardening. I discovered that getting my hands in the soil gave me a strong connection with the earth, making me feel a part of the earth, the womb from which I had come. The earth nourished me with her food as I grew in my mother's womb, and it has continued to give me sustenance throughout the years. During my pregnancy, as soon as the ground was dry enough to work after the heavy California rains, I spread a winter's worth of compost over last year's vegetable garden. As I watched my husband till the compost into the soil, the earth became even more alive as if rejuvenated by the nourishment that was given her. Getting my hands into the soil while planting the tomato or squash felt so right.

Gardening is very rewarding and simple, whether you choose to start a vegetable or flower garden. To plant a seed and watch it grow is a miracle quite comparable, of course, to the seed growing inside the womb. Even those living in an apartment can grow house plants or go to a place where one can do some gardening. Working with the earth has helped to "center" me and to make me feel stronger about myself.

I heat my house with wood and enjoy cutting the dead trees on my property that provide heat for my house. I love walking through the woods, finding the dead trees, cutting them up, and hauling them home. I like stacking the logs neatly on a pile to dry thoroughly for the next winter. This process makes me feel whole and empowered, for I am able to provide one of life's most basic necessities—warmth—for myself and my family. In addition, I don't have to pay any heating bills or anyone else to deliver the wood. Besides, it gets me out in nature, breathing the fresh air and listening to the songs of the birds and the wind rustling through the trees, reminding me of the part I play in the whole planetary scheme.

While in nature, whether in the woods or in a park, I find solace and reassurance in watching the insects and the animals whose lives are so simple compared to many of our own. They need only the basics, and they appear to be content with that. Being in nature while pregnant reminds us of where our roots lie buried. It also helps us get in touch with the womanly spirit—that record of millions of years of the female experience encoded in our DNA on how to intuitively give birth with ecstasy. When an animal gives birth, complications seldom arise. This natural process takes place on its own without much interference, except maybe from a predator. And if a predator or danger does appear, the animal's labor will stop, giving her time to flee. Perhaps it is the fear that sends the hormones racing through her blood stream, a fear that might be similar to the fear experienced by women while in labor when their labor slows or stops altogether.

Society sometimes feeds on the fears and insecurities of women. For example, once a woman announces that she is pregnant, she automatically belongs to society; she no longer is quite her own person. Friends, relatives, the old lady on the bus—all well wishers—think nothing of offering advice on what to do during pregnancy and birth. Some will adamantly condemn homebirths, and at the mention of water births, all hell can break loose. So before making any "rebel" declarations, a woman should consider her audience and not feel compelled to go into full detail of how she intends to give birth. Some may react negatively out of ignorance, but others only out of concern for you and the baby. Especially when a woman is making decisions that are controversial, she needs positive support to withstand the orthodoxy of doctors who have strong ideas about what is the normal and the best way to be pregnant and have a baby.

As all pregnant women will tell you, they will be bombarded with other people's birth stories or stories of their pregnancies. While it is completely natural to want to speak about one's labor and delivery, which, after all is one of the most incredible experiences of a lifetime, when the horror stories begin to unfold, the expectant mom should make a quick excuse and remove herself from the conversation. In a society that fears pregnancy and birth, no one needs to be subjected to more anxieties while pregnant.

EDUCATION

To get the most out of her pregnancy and birth experience, a woman needs to make informed decisions. And to make informed decisions, she needs to be educated about pregnancy, labor, delivery, and the postpartum period. She should read as many books as possible about the changes that the pregnant body is going through, as well as the developmental stages of the fetus. It is especially important for women to understand what their bodies are doing while in labor, for this knowledge will help lessen the likelihood that they will succumb to fear. Both mother and father should be well educated about labor and delivery, so that in the event of complications, the best decisions will be made. Part of obtaining good prenatal care is educating oneself on matters one doesn't understand.

Attending childbirth classes is one way to get this education. Classes are very important for pregnant couples simply because in this way they can be exposed to others with similar questions and feelings. Classes are of particular importance for the fathers, since they themselves are not physically pregnant and so may not understand what the mother is going through physiologically, emotionally, and spiritually. In addition, the fathers may need some emotional support themselves and may find that other fathers are having similar questions and feelings. A childbirth class can also be a very supportive environment in which to ask what may appear to be stupid questions. It is always surprising how many others have similar questions. As for the mothers, being around people who want similar things for their babies and themselves can lessen their feelings of being alone in their decision against a hospital birth. Group support is always helpful in this case.

Finding the *right* childbirth class is important. For example, those who want homebirth classes will feel very uncomfortable in a class with people preparing for hospital births. Usually, the Bradley method offers classes that are oriented toward natural childbirth, and there is a better chance of getting together with other people who want a homebirth. The Bradley method is also preferable because of the type of breathing that is taught. It is a deep abdominal breathing that helps the mother relax.

As stated in an earlier chapter, it is preferable to take classes from the person who is going to be your midwife. If that is not possible, perhaps the midwife can recommend a class that will be suitable for someone wanting a homebirth or a water birth.

The topics that should be included in childbirth class are the different stages of labor, including what to expect and what complications can arise at each stage; exercises, for both toning up the body and relaxation; a synopsis of the anatomy and physiology of pregnancy and labor, as well as the developmental stages of the fetus; nutrition and herbs; what to expect if one has to go to the hospital and what drugs are used; breastfeeding and care for the mother and newborn; and watching videos and slides of women giving birth. I ask anyone who is going to be at the birth to view these films and slides, which never fail to leave people in awe. The old saying, "A picture is worth a thousand words," is indeed true. Just seeing the videos can put the mind at ease and bring up questions that can be answered in class, alleviating many potential fears and trepidations. It is particularly important for people having a water birth to see as many videos and slides as possible and to invite any one who is going to be present at the birth to view them as well. Igor Charkowsky advises that for anyone who is going to be involved with the birth, including the mother and father, some attention should be paid to alleviating fears beforehand. Once those involved with the birth have viewed the videos, all are convinced of the simplicity and wonderful advantages of water for both mother and baby.

Couples desiring a water birth should speak with couples who have already had a water birth. It is very reassuring to find others who have successfully attempted this approach to giving birth. It is also great to meet the children who were born in that milieu, to see that they are fine, healthy individuals who have had a good start in life.

I also recommend books to the couples that I work with for information on nutrition, childbirth, water birth, breastfeeding, and other topics. These books are an important part of their education. There are also many more books available that will be fun and informative. The books are listed in the Suggested Readings.

NUTRITION

Good nutrition is crucial for the mother's health and the baby's development. Good nutrition makes the mother happier and gives her a positive frame of mind, which makes an important imprint on the growing fetus.

Ideally, the woman has been preparing for the conception of the baby by eating good healthy foods, participating in an exercise program, and learning to alleviate stress through meditation or various other methods of relaxation. The mother's body not only houses her soul, but is also the vehicle through which the baby's body is nourished and developed. Therefore, the mother's body should be free from the toxins accumulated through drinking alcohol, smoking, prescription and nonprescription drugs, food, and the air—all can contribute to an unhealthy body.

Fasting before conception will start releasing the toxins; then both mother and father should begin eating a diet free from chemicals and high in organic foods. Remember, this is recommended as the ideal, the goal. Don't chastise yourself if you are unable to plan your conception. Most of us would not be here if our parents had planned our coming.

Once the mother knows she is pregnant, she can start cutting out foods that are not beneficial and start adding organic foods that will promote health for mother, father, and the growing baby. She should start by eliminating foods that are refined or processed (stripped of their natural state), or any foods containing chemical additives or preservatives. These chemicals may be teratogenic and carcinogenic. Read all labels on packages. Foods with preservatives are not fresh, or why else would these be added, except to prolong shelf life? Buy whole grains and foods that have been grown organically. Not only will they be healthier for mother and baby, but also they will taste better. If you eat meat, try to cut down on red meat, or find a source for beef that is raised organically. Now that there is a consumer demand for it, it is becoming easier to find meat that has been raised organically. Please do not convert to a vegetarian diet while pregnant or nursing. Such a change in diet can trigger the body into releasing toxins that would go directly to the baby.

A favorite book of mine—one that I used during my own pregnancy—contains good guidelines for healthy foods for pregnant women. Paavo Airola's *Every Woman's Book* (1979) will help you nurture the growing child and to live healthfully through the different phases of womanhood.

I ask the pregnant women whom I instruct to keep a journal of what they eat over a one- to two-week period. I check the journal several times during the course of the prenatal care to get an idea of how they are eating and also to remind them to eat well-balanced meals.

Most midwives believe it is important to help the mother maintain her blood count (hematocrit and hemoglobin) at an optimum range. As noted earlier, I do not feel comfortable attending a water birth when the mother's hematocrit is under 36 or the hemoglobin is under 12. It is not safe. Since the red blood cells are the oxygen carriers, the infant will not receive sufficient amounts of oxygen through the umbilical cord unless the hematocrit and hemoglobin are in a safe range. A higher hematocrit and hemoglobin also lessens the likelihood that the mother will hemorrhage, and if she does, it will be less traumatic for her body if she should lose more than the average amount of blood.

Local health food stores usually carry good organic prenatal vitamins, or the birth attendant may be able to recommend good nutritional supplements. Those having problems getting their blood count up should ask their birth attendant to recommend a good chelated iron. This iron is easier to assimilate and is less constipating. Many women have told me of an iron and herb liquid extract that they used to get the iron up. It is called Floradix and is made in Germany. It is obtained through Miracle Exclusive, Locust Valley, New York 11560. I have seen amazing results with this extract, and women have informed me that their energy level seems to increase when they are taking it.

Women have also told me that eating foods high in iron has helped keep their iron levels up. A good resource to learn about foods high in iron is a book called *Composition and Facts About Foods,* by Ford Heritage (1971). Vegetables high in iron include green leafy vegetables like spinach, red chard, red leaf lettuce, beets and beet greens, dulse, kelp, pumpkin, and squash seeds, whole sesame seeds, wheat germ, sunflower seeds and sprouts, parsley, and dried fruits.

One woman claimed that two tablespoons of blackstrap molasses (the unsulphured kind, of course) in an 8-ounce glass of milk two times a day helps to increase her iron count. Several other women have tried this regimen with winning results.

Yet another woman told me of herbs such as yellow dock (*Rumex crispus*) and stinging nettle (*Urtica dioica*), which can be drunk as a tea or made into tinctures, both of which are very high in iron. Other teas also appear to be helpful during pregnancy. For example, red raspberry (*Rubus strigosus*) has been traditional for generations among Native American women as a uterine toner. It is also said to be high in iron. I drank two to three cups daily during my pregnancy, and I had a quick and easy labor. I am not saying that drinking these teas will ensure an easy labor, but several women have told me that they felt a difference in the efficiency of the contractions during labor when they drank the tea with one pregnancy as compared to another pregnancy when they didn't drink it. Comfrey (*Symphytum officinale*) is high in amino acids that help assimilate proteins for building strong muscles. It is also high in iron and calcium. This herb is controversial, however, with some claiming it to be carcinogenic, although not all authorities agree. Comfrey should therefore be used with discretion. Other herbs high in calcium are borage (*Borage offficinalis*), dandelion root (*Taraxacum officinale*), stinging nettle (*Urtica dioica*), horsetail (*Equesteum arvense*), and red clover (*Trifolium pratense*).

A woman herbalist told me that during her eighth month of pregnancy she drank Shepherd's Purse tea (*Capsella Bursa-pastoris*) in addition to red raspberry (*Rubis strigosus*) tea. She informed me that Shepherd's Purse is high in vitamin K, which is a blood coagulant and can help prevent hemorrhaging. It can be made into a tincture along with another herb high in vitamin K, alfalfa (*Medicago sativa*), or the two can be made into a tea. She felt that the vitamin K would also get to the fetus through the mother, therefore giving the newborn a jumpstart on the assimilation of the vitamin. *Please consult with your physician or midwife before using these herbs.*

Most people do not drink enough water. During pregnancy, it is important to drink as much water as possible—at least two liters of water a day. Some people groan at the thought of drinking so much water while being pregnant. "I'll have to be running to the bathroom every ten minutes!" one woman exclaimed. But keeping the body well hydrated is important, because flushing the system with water helps to get toxins out of the mother's body, therefore keeping the fetus in a healthier state. During pregnancy the body is producing more water, and therefore the source needs to be replenished. Keeping fluids in the body also helps with the production of breast milk.

I instruct the mothers to get two quart jars and fill them with water every morning. Their goal is to have finished the jars before they go to bed. The teas can be sipped in between times.

As for food cravings, we wouldn't be human if we didn't have them. I believe it is fine to give into them occasionally, as long as the intake of junk food is not a daily affair.

I recall one mother who probably was on the strictest and healthiest diet I had ever seen. I laugh when I think of coming upon her in a restaurant, with her beaming eyes and her big belly of nine months, sitting behind a mound of whipped cream, hot fudge, and three big scoops of ice cream. Her jaw dropped, and her eyes bugged out when she saw me, thinking she had been caught by her midwife doing something wrong. I loved it! I was glad to see her feeling so good and so happy just from eating a hot fudge sundae. It was probably doing her a world of good to indulge herself occasionally rather than always denying herself.

EXERCISE

Exercise and relaxation are essential for a healthy pregnancy and birth. Preparing oneself physically is important not only for the pregnancy and birth, but also for the time after the baby is born. Restoring the muscles, ligaments, joints, and tissues to their former shape will help develop a body that will work well for the rest of one's life. And, too, if the body is physically in shape, the hormones will have an easier time balancing themselves throughout all the shifts that occur in pregnancy. According to Elizabeth Noble, "The process is like giving a party. . . . The actual event seems to pass quickly because we are excited and preoccupied. After the party is over, there's a lot more work to be done before the house gets back into shape and working order again" (1982, p. 1). I highly recommend Noble's book for its well-rounded examples of exercises and information on how the body works during the perinatal period.

When it comes to exercise, I believe that swimming, walking, and stretching (hatha yoga) are physically beneficial, and also contribute to relaxation and proper breathing. If these exercises can be done in the sunshine and fresh air, then they are doubly beneficial.

For those already involved in aerobic exercise, studies have shown that aerobic exercise may be continued as long as any warning signs are noted. A study published in the *Journal of Nurse-Midwifery* by Sibley et al. (1981) states that

> ideally a woman would be in good physical condition prior to pregnancy, but if not, she may begin a program of progressive exercise provided there are no prior health indications. . . . Women should begin any aerobic exercise program gently, building strength and endurance slowly over time. This is important not only to accustom the heart and lungs to new demands, but also to allow the joints, tendons, and muscles to adjust themselves to the new activity. During exercise, it is important that a woman be aware of such symptoms of overexertion as tightness or pain in the chest, severe breathlessness, lightheadedness, dizziness, headache, loss of muscle control, and nausea. If any of these symptoms appear, exercise should be stopped immediately. . . . It is important to appropriately in-

crease calories, fluids, and rest to cover energy expenditures; and to obtain prenatal care throughout pregnancy (p. 9).

The study goes on to say that "The data obtained from the exercise tests suggest that it is possible to safely maintain physical fitness by regular participation in aerobic exercise during pregnancy" (p. 9).

Swimming

My work with Igor Charkowsky confirmed the importance of swimming while pregnant. The pregnant mothers who followed his advice on swimming preparations were very fit and toned, and most gave birth with ease in the squatting position. Access to swimming pools is fairly easy in Moscow, and so Charkowsky instructs women to swim daily. Despite the abundance of indoor pools, in the dead of winter pregnant women can be seen swimming outdoors, which they believe strengthens them physically and psychologically for enduring labor. Swimming is a family event, with the fathers and children swimming side by side with the pregnant moms. Little children not yet able to walk freely swim above and below the water as if they were amphibious creatures.

Along with swimming laps, swimming under water for set periods of time increases the lung capacity in preparation for childbirth. The movements women make under water help to strengthen crucial areas of the body to help support a growing belly and to maintain the muscles used while squatting to give birth. Tanya, one of the midwives who works with Charkowsky, practiced doing the dolphin's movements while under water. The motions in the water helped to strengthen her lower back and abdominal muscles, muscles that can undergo a lot of strain during pregnancy and afterward need toning. Tanya would meditate under water. Crossing her legs and putting each foot on the opposite thigh (in the full lotus position), Tanya would float in the water with arms extended or hold her nose to prevent water from getting in. Meditating in water was important, she explained, for it put the body in a completely relaxed state due to reduced gravity. The mother should also try to envision what it is like to be a fetus in the womb, remembering what it felt like to be inside her own mother. Tanya would also do twirling motions while in water, which worked to strengthen her back muscles.

In the style of the Polar Bear clubs in the United States, pregnant women working with Charkowsky would jump into water through holes in the ice, swim around for a few seconds and come out again. This activity would be repeated several times. It was quite a contrast to see the elderly women, wearing their babushkas and bundled snuggly in the background looking on at the young women in their bikinis with their fig-shaped bodies jumping in and out of the freezing water. These immersions gave them mental strength and endurance, both of which are crucial when laboring. Observing them was like watching athletes preparing for the big event.

Charkowsky believes that swimming is an excellent way to "connect" with the baby, meaning to be able to feel what the baby feels, to be able to converse psychically with the unborn child, to acquire empathetic feelings of what it feels like to be in water. Because we came from the water—and indeed are made mostly of water—we can relax and allow its buoyancy to release our stress, creating a more peaceful environment for the growing child within.

I can remember that wonderful feeling of weightlessness while swimming during my ninth month of pregnancy. Out of the water I felt so huge; in the water I felt I had lost all the extra weight and was light again. Even my low back pain disappeared.

Swimming also helps to strengthen important muscles needed to help carry the baby during pregnancy and to give tone to the body afterward. Most important, the body is in shape to give birth to the baby. I sometimes felt as if I was preparing for an endurance test, even a triathalon. It felt so great to be physically fit.

Walking

Walking can be a real treat. It gets us out of the house and often gives us a different perspective on things. A brisk walk in the fresh air helps to strengthen those leg muscles that need to be strong for squatting while giving birth. A few women have told me that taking a walk with their partners was one of the few times they could be alone with them and get their full attention. When teaching childbirth classes, I remind the men that the walks are an important part of the exercise program. Sometimes I hear groans from the tired-looking men, who seem to be saying: "Isn't working hard all day enough? All I want to do is come home and rest. It is the last thing that I want to do is get up and go for a walk!" It's at this point that I hand out the reminder cards that say, "Taking care of the mother is taking care of your child."

If no other form of exercise can be done, walking is an easy way of getting into shape; it is also a nice time to check in with each other to see how "we" are doing. In the ninth month of pregnancy, walking is essential, for it assists in lowering the baby deeper into the birth canal, helping the baby's head to engage. With the head engaged, there is less work for both baby and mother once labor begins. This means a shorter and less tiring labor for both. Some good strong walking for a mile may be essential when a first-time mom is thirty-eight weeks into the gestation and the baby's head has not yet engaged. Stopping periodically on the walk and doing some squatting helps to lower the head into the birth canal. Walking around the block a few times or through a park will suffice if it is impossible to get to the country.

Yoga/Stretching

Yoga or stretching integrates body, mind, spirit, and breath. It also helps the body to relax and, if done correctly, to stretch to its fullest potential. The deep abdominal breathing used during the yoga postures is the same breathing rhythms used during the early stages of labor.

I highly recommend Jeanine Parvati Baker's book *Prenatal Yoga and Natural Birth* (1974). This book, though now twenty years old, remains an excellent source for prenatal exercise for thousands of women. Particularly good are the cat stretch and the dog tail wag exercises. I like this book because the exercises are simple and effective, and can be done by almost everyone.

Another very informative book is Janet Balaskas's *New Active Birth* (1993). It includes helpful information for the entire perinatal period. It is full of stretching exercises that produce amazing results for women who have lost the strength and tone in the muscles that are necessary for squatting or supporting the back and abdomen. I didn't use these exercises when I was pregnant because I did not know about them. Later on, I became friends with Janet's sister-in-law, Meloma Balaskas, who at the time lived in Berkeley. Often upon arriving at her home, she would answer the door by asking, "Want to have a stretch?" Looking in the room, I would see half a dozen women with their feet and legs up on the wall, chatting away as if sitting at a table and having a tea. The stretching felt very beneficial in all the right places for the women preparing for birth and the postpartum period.

Over time, these slow and easy stretches strengthen the muscles necessary for birth (and some of the unnecessary ones too). Several of the women had previously given birth and noted how they did not have the low back pain they had experienced in other pregnancies. These classes were such fun, but unfortunately Meloma lived over an hour's drive so that I could not come to her classes very often.

THE KEGEL MUSCLE

The Kegel muscle, simply put, is the muscle we use to stop ourselves from urinating while standing in the grocery line. It is very important to exercise this muscle early in pregnancy, and you will be glad you did for years after your baby is born. Strengthening this particular muscle helps with bladder control during the last months of the pregnancy when the baby's head feels as if it is bouncing up and down on the

Figure 1
The Kegel Muscle

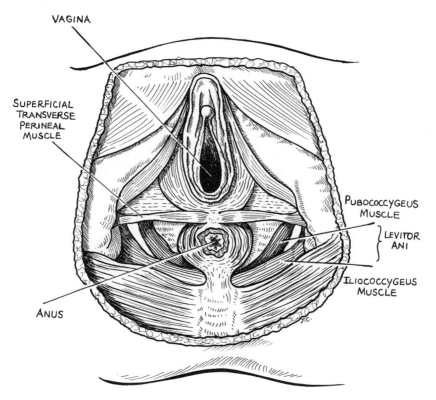

VAGINA

SUPERFICIAL
TRANSVERSE
PERINEAL
MUSCLE

PUBOCOCCYGEUS
MUSCLE

} LEVITOR
  ANI

ILIOCOCCYGEUS
MUSCLE

ANUS

Figure by Jeff Cox

bladder. Kegel exercises can be done discreetly anywhere, at any time. In my childbirth classes, I instruct both moms and dads to locate the muscle that they use to stop urinating midflow. I ask them to visualize this muscle as an elevator in a department store going from the basement floor to the sixth floor. The elevator (the Kegel muscle) goes up to the first floor and stops. Hold that muscle as people need to get on and off of the elevator. Go up to the second floor and hold that muscle tight on the second floor for a while to once again let the people on and off. Slowly, do this up to the sixth floor, and then slowly bring it back down in the same manner. In this way, the Kegel muscle is slowly being tightened, held, and then released. This exercise strengthens the muscle for good bladder control. So many women regret not doing this exercise and complain that even years after having a baby occasionally when they sneeze hard, they will wet their pants.

PERINEAL MASSAGE

The perineum is the tissue and skin between the anus and the vaginal opening. This skin stretches like a turtleneck sweater around the baby's head as he emerges from the vagina. The head pops out, rotates, allowing the shoulders and the rest of the baby's body to emerge. The perineum can be massaged prior to the head showing as well as when the head is emerging, which puts the pressure on the perineum. The massage helps keep the blood circulating in the tissue so that the tissue remains elastic and stretches well while the head is coming through. In hospitals, the perineum is routinely cut, unless the parents request otherwise ahead of time. Once cut, the perineum needs to be stitched back up again. The doctors in the hospitals cut the perineum to prevent tearing, assuming that the perineum automatically tears. Many women tell me that they have no discomfort after the birth except for the stitches in the perineum.

I have witnessed hundreds of women who slowly pushed their babies out while getting their perineums massaged and supported. The tissue slowly stretches. I seldom see a tear—maybe a few skid marks but nothing serious. Most of these women prepare themselves months ahead of time by oiling their perineums and vaginal floors and slowly pressing down, while sliding their fingers around the opening of the vagina. (Wheat germ oil or a nonviscous vitamin E oil helps to nourish the skin.) The woman's partner can also do this for her, slowly stretching the skin more and more. One can start with one or two fingers and throughout the months put more fingers into the vagina as the area stretches more willingly. Remember, a baby's head must fit through there, so do not be afraid to stretch it. Lovemaking is also a good way to stretch the perineal area, if it is not done too forcefully. While birthing in the water, the warm water helps the skin to stretch more than giving birth on a bed. However, it is important to be aware of the possibility of the tissue tearing, especially when delivering large babies. Remember that nature makes no guarantees.

BREATHING

Most of us have forgotten how to breathe with our full lung capacity. Our lungs are protected by our rib cage and fill approximately three-quarters of the rib area. Most of us breathe very shallowly, using only our upper lungs and neglecting our middle and lower lungs. Therefore, our blood is not as well oxygenated as it could be. Using our full lung capacity is even more important during the perinatal time, pregnancy, labor, and nursing.

As we all know, the mother's blood supplies the oxygen to the fetus;

therefore, breathing with all the lung area is important for the development of the fetus. This is even more important in labor because the baby may be getting stressed as a result of the contractions and the descent of the head through the birth canal. This is the time that the fetus needs to be well oxygenated, so that if a problem does arise, the fetus will have less chance of oxygen deprivation.

The nursing mother needs the oxygen to help with the milk supply, as well as to get enough oxygen to her tissues, muscles, joints, and bones so that they are able to return to their former shape.

During my childbirth classes, I give several sessions on correct breathing. Believe it or not, breathing takes practice. For many of us, we have not breathed properly since childhood. I invite the couples to sit on the floor, the pregnant women sitting cross-legged (some would call this Indian fashion) and their partners or labor coaches sitting on the floor behind them. The partners' hands are placed on either side of the rib cage just below the women's breasts. The women pretend that their lungs are bellows and try to push away their partner's hands with their rib cage. During this motion, the women's shoulders are not to move up. The goal is to breathe with our diaphragms and use our full lung capacity. If the shoulders start moving up, then the exercise is being done incorrectly; the shoulders need to remain still. Another way to practice breathing is to lie on the floor and put a book over one's diaphragm. While breathing, the book should be moved up and down. Try doing this every day, from as early in the pregnancy as possible. And, of course, exercise performed in fresh air and sunshine contribute to health and vitality.

MEDITATION AND VISUALIZATION

Meditation during pregnancy is important simply because in the frenetic world we live in we have to take some time out to quiet our minds and relax. Even if done only once a day for half an hour, noticeable results will be visible. Being more relaxed and calmer are two benefits to begin with. Through meditation I found that I was able to let go of the stress that is the unfortunate price we pay to live in the "civilized" world. I felt able to reclaim my body and to touch base with my intuitive rhythms.

If you enjoy doing your exercises or meditations outdoors, you will be reaping even more benefits. The sun and fresh air are very beneficial to both mother's and baby's health. Being in nature is a positive factor for any woman. The earth is the mother giving us strength and helping us to connect with our womanhood and our instinctive knowledge of birth. Spending time with the earth helps maintain our connection with our female ancestors who worked so closely with the land. These women did not bury their female knowledge of the ways of Mother Earth, such as so many of us have had to do in order to blend into the industrialized world. Many women, forced to depend on artificial and misconstrued help in order to give birth, see fewer and fewer examples in our day-to-day lives of what being a mother is about.

Some psychologists believe that the baby is able to feel the feelings that the mother feels, whether emotional or physical. Some also believe that the mother can communicate with her baby on a psychic level and know what the baby is feeling. Almost every pregnant mother I have worked with, at some time during her pregnancy, has felt that she could feel what the fetus felt or that the fetus would communicate with her.

Part of caring for your baby and yourself prenatally is to sit quietly and send love to the baby. Talk to the baby. Rub your belly and see how your baby responds. In response they sometimes kick or wiggle around.

A nice meditation the couple can do together is to sit calmly and face each other. In your mind's eye, picture a triangle connecting the mother, father, and baby. Picture your baby in your mind. Look at the different parts of the body, the little feet with the little toes and the hands that will someday hold yours; your baby's sweet face and sweet smile. Then imagine how wonderful it will be to hold that baby in your arms. Send your baby all the love that is in both of your hearts—a total unconditional love respecting who that individual is. Imagine that the baby is actually present with you on the outside of your body. Lennart Nilsson's *A Child Is Born* (1977) helps couples visualize the baby's different developmental stages in a striking series of photographs.

This exercise is important for several reasons: in our too-busy lives, it is easy to let the months slip by and the pregnancy is gone. Doing this exercise makes the parents sit down and not only take time out for themselves, but also to concentrate on this new person that is soon to be such a big part of their lives. The meditation acknowledges the baby and gives the baby recognition. It also gets the father involved. He may feel alienated during the pregnancy because he is not physically involved with the incubation process; through this meditation, he can feel involved and be spiritually connected. At the end of the meditation, the parents may want to say a closing prayer or perform a ritual that feels pleasing.

Visualizations and Affirmations

I am a strong proponent of visualizations and affirmations simply because I have seen them work so well during labor and delivery. These strong mental tools may be simply described as mind over matter. I encourage pregnant women to use visualizations to establish an in utero communication with the baby, an exercise that I have previously explained. A visualization is picturing in one's mind what one wants to see accomplished, whereas an affirmation is making positive reinforcing statements to oneself in conjunction with the visualizations. For example, during my pregnancy I tried to see myself as a strong lioness. I kept reminding myself of the Native American women who would go off in the woods by themselves or assisted by a midwife, just squat down on the earth, or hang on to a tree for support, and give birth to the baby with such strength and power. I kept telling myself that I would have an easy birth. I had no doubts about giving birth at home or in the water. I had seen both work many times. I would visualize in my mind everything that I wanted to happen at my son's birth, but from my professional experience, I knew that nature makes no guarantees. Birth does not always go the way one wants it to go; nonetheless, these exercises are helpful.

As it turned out, I had a very difficult pregnancy. I bled for two weeks during my fourth month and had to stay in bed. I was terrified of losing my baby, and yet I was bound and determined to keep the baby in me. I kept my hand on my abdomen while talking to the baby, telling him how much I loved him and how much I wanted him to stay with me. I visualized a strong healthy placenta attaching itself firmly to the wall of my uterus. I visualized my baby as strong and healthy, happy to be growing inside of me. I told him what fun we would have together after he was born and growing into a man. I firmly believe this all helped. I was able to keep my son in me, even though every doctor and midwife told me to be prepared for the worst. During my labor I used my visualizations, thinking of the infinite lineage of women who have given birth since the beginning of time. So I gave birth with the strength of a lioness. No, everything did not go the way I wanted it to go, but the strength and power that I felt when I pushed my baby through was the culmination of all those women who have given birth since the beginning of time. I could have moved mountains.

MASSAGE

It is no wonder that a cat purrs when being petted; it feels really good to be touched. Americans do not touch enough, mainly because of all our cultural biases about touching and showing affection. Getting massages is a wonderful way to relax muscles that are deep in the body that may have been tense for years. Having worked as a professional masseuse, I am amazed at the minute number of people who do not have tight muscles—who are not carrying around a lot of stress in their bodies. Sometimes we have to help our muscles to remember how to relax. Through massage we are retraining them. For a pregnant woman it is essential that her muscles be taught to relax so that she can let loose and let her baby come through while in labor. I can remember a woman whose thighs and buttocks muscles were so tight while in labor that they felt like bands of steel. These muscles are some of the most important ones to relax, allowing dilation to take place and the baby to move out. Most women's muscles would respond to massage while in labor, but this woman's muscles didn't. After the birth she claimed that her area of greatest stress was in her thighs and buttocks. If she had been getting massages during her pregnancy, these muscles would have been trained to relax and would have responded to massage more easily.

In the ideal, the pregnant mother should get a massage once a week; if that is not affordable, then possibly twice a month or once a month will do. The partner of the pregnant woman can always give her a massage, which may be a good opportunity for the two of them to take time out for each other and enjoy each other's company. A full body massage is best with emphasis on the inner and outer thighs and the buttocks to teach these areas to stretch and relax. Pregnant mothers usually enjoy footrubs and backrubs. *Please do not rub the ankles and the calves, for these areas have points in the body that connect to the uterus and cervix and could possibly put the mother into premature labor.*

PRENATAL VISITS WITH YOUR DOCTOR OR MIDWIFE

When the couple and the midwife come to a decision to work together, it is important for the midwife to give a written statement of policy. This document states what the couple can expect of her, how she practices, and what she expects of the couple. Each midwife should present this policy to the couple so that the couple will have exact knowledge of the midwife's own individual boundaries for her practice and not have expectations that exceed what the midwife can give. In the event of any misunderstandings, the couple and midwife will have clear and ready access to guidelines on how they can work together.

I tell every couple that the ultimate outcome of a birth is a healthy mother and baby and that, if complications arise, I may stop the couple from having a water birth, and encourage them to discontinue proceeding with laboring or birthing in the water. They may be able to continue with a homebirth, or, if necessary, go to the hospital. It is important not to be so attached to one particular method that the chief goal—a healthy mother and baby—is forgotten.

The midwife should get together with the couples at least once a month for their prenatal visits until the eighth month, when they should see each other every two weeks. In the ninth month, they should get together every week until the baby is born. These are the same time intervals recommended by an obstetrician in every standard practice in the United States.

On the initial visit, the mother's medical history, as well as her immediate family history and the father's, is taken. This history may alert the midwife to problems that may evolve during the pregnancy or problems that the baby may have. For example, the midwife should know if the pregnant mother's grandmother had twins, or if there are a lot of allergies on both the maternal and paternal sides of the baby's family.

I allot about one hour for each prenatal visit. During this time, I try to get to know the couple, to assess their relationship, and to perceive the stress level in their life; I also want them to get to know me. It is important that people feel comfortable and trust each other. The pregnancy and birth are very intimate times during the couple's life. The midwife and the couples become very close during the pregnancy. When the baby is born and the postpartum care is completed, however, the midwife and the couple are usually not as in close contact with each other, for new priorities are now in place. One new mother likened the bittersweet conclusion to losing a lover, because of the bonding that takes place. This bonding, of course, does not always occur, but when it does, it makes for a better relationship for all involved.

To encourage couples to be involved with their own prenatal care, I insist that the father or partner be present at each session. I also instruct the father to do the prenatal care, and I check his results.

At every visit the pregnant mother's blood pressure is taken, the baby's heartbeat is checked with a fetoscope, and the baby's growth is recorded by measuring the fundal height (measuring from the top of the pubic arch to the top of the uterus). The abdomen is also palpated to see what position the baby is lying in. A urine sample is taken to test with reagent strips for protein and sugar in the urine. The Ph may also be taken if the couple so desires. All of this can be taught to the father and the mother and, for double security, can be checked over by the midwife. Fathers usually love to get involved, for it makes them feel they are part of the pregnancy.

Nutrition should be discussed at every visit. Periodically, I ask the pregnant mother to give me a menu of what she eats and drinks for two weeks. This means everything including water and what quantity she consumes. I want to know if she is having any discomforts, headache, nausea, swelling, or anything in the slightest that may be a problem.

Approximately every two months the pregnant mother's blood is checked, especially for the hematocrit and hemoglobin. Both of these tests are included in a CBC (complete blood count and differential), a series of tests of the peripheral blood that give information about the hemotologic system and a few other organ systems. The tests can be done quickly and somewhat inexpensively. Included in the tests are red blood cell count (RBC), hemoglobin (Hgb), and hematocrit (HCt). Red blood cell indices include mean corpuscular volume (MCV), mean corpuscular hemoglobin (MCH), and mean corpuscular hemoglobin concentration (MCHC). Also included are white blood cell count (WBC) and differential count, neurtrophis (polynucleated cells), Basophils, Lymphocytes, Eosinophis, and Monocytes. The CBC also includes a blood smear and a platelet count.

I also ask the pregnant mother to have her blood typed if she does not already know what it is. If she has not had German measles, she also needs to have a rubella antibody test (German measles test). The Hct and Hgb can be done separately from a CBC if additional tests need to be done periodically to screen for anemia. I require an HIV test in the ninth month of pregnancy because when working with water births, the midwife may have to get into the water in an emergency. In addition, the baby may need special care at birth if the mother is HIV positive and may need to go to or be born in the hospital. Good books for deciphering lab work are *Mosby's Diagnostic and Laboratory Test Reference* by Kathleen Pagana and Timothy Pagana (1992) and *Understanding Lab Work in the Childbearing Year* by Anne Frye (1990).

REASONS FOR REFUSING A COUPLE FOR A WATER BIRTH

Rarely do I feel uncomfortable with people. Occasionally, on the first meeting I do not feel that working with the couple may be right. This may also happen later on in the pregnancy when something just doesn't feel right. If I follow my intuition, I usually get confirming evidence that I was right. Sometimes the couple will feel the same way.

Sometimes, contraindications may show up during the pregnancy that indicate that the mother should go to the hospital instead of proceeding with a traditional homebirth. Most of the "signals" that alert me are the same as those that I would use for any homebirth. These contraindications may be:

1. Becoming an insulin-dependent diabetic.
2. Significant cardiac conditions.
3. Unwillingness or inability to follow my criteria for prenatal care and birth preparation.
4. Former cephalopelvic disproportion due to mother's skeletal structure.
5. Inadequate home environment. (This could mean a variety of things, depending on the midwife's standards. For instance, one couple was

having problems with their well, and upon having the water tested, they found that the water was full of E coli. They said they had it cleared up, but when the tank was filling, I looked at the water and found it to be very muddy. I did not feel that the water was clean enough for a woman to give birth in safely. An adequate heat source in the house is also needed in order to maintain a temperature of at least 70° F. There should also be electricity, so that a constant temperature can be maintained in the birthing tank. And needless to say, a clean house is a must.

6. Over forty-five minutes to an emergency facility either by car or helicopter.

7. Eclampsia.

8. Outbreak of herpes while in labor.

9. Low hematocrit and hemoglobin.

10. Multiple pregnancy. (I personally do not feel comfortable with working with twins in water simply because I have not attempted it. I have known of a very successful birth of twins in water in Oregon.)

11. Breech presentations. It is up to the midwife to decide if she feels competent to attend a breech. Whether birth takes place on a bed or in the water, breech presentations are always tricky.

12. Low-lying placenta covering os.

13. Infectious diseases that can be transferred by water, such as strep and staph.

14. Inability to obtain required supplies for homebirth and water birth.

15. Dogmatic disposition of the couple to have a water birth at all costs.

16. People who want pain killers while in labor, heavy smokers, drug users, or heavy alcohol drinkers.

ITEMS NEEDED FOR A HOMEBIRTH AND A WATER BIRTH

1. *Plastic drop cloth or shower curtain.* This is to protect the mattress that the mother labors on from anything that may get it wet. The labor bed can be made up as follows: on the very bottom of the mattress is a clean set of sheets that the mother can get into after the baby is born. The plastic drop cloth is placed on top of these sheets to keep the sheets clean and free from getting wet. On top of the drop cloth go the sterilized sheets (see #21) for laboring on.

2. *Tincture of green soap.* This soap is used for washing hands or any items that may need to be scrubbed before use during labor or afterward.

3. *Betadine solution or scrub.* Sometimes as much as a liter of betadine is needed for several uses. One of the main purposes is to scrub out the tank before adding the water that the mother is to labor in. I

also ask anyone who gets into the tank to shower before getting into the tank, using the betadine instead of soap. It is also put in the footbath. (I will describe this later in the list.)

4. *Unopened bottle of oil for perineal massage* (Olive oil will do). The bottle needs to remain sealed to keep the oil from contamination. This oil is needed in case it becomes impossible to proceed with a water birth. The oil is not used in the water.

5. *Disposable underpads—Durasorbs or Chux.* This is for added protection while laboring on the bed in case the bag of waters should break, or some blood or feces should come out; then the whole sheet does not have to be changed. I prefer using the disposable underpads instead of towels.

6. *Hospital-size modess and belt.* Get at least two boxes. They need to be changed every hour or so. Tampons should never be worn after delivery because they can cause a severe infection.

7. *Infant ear syringe* (3- or 4-ounce size only please). This is for cleaning out the air passages of the newborn and should be kept close by for the first week or so.

8. *An umbilical clamp or white cotton shoe laces.* This is for clamping off the umbilical cord after it has been cut.

9. *Cotton balls.* Or just plain sterile cotton that is used for dabbing alcohol on the stump of the baby's umbilical cord to ward off infections.

10. *Gauze pads.* Twenty or more individually wrapped, sterile. These are used during the birth or afterward for many different functions.

11. *Enema equipment.* Women have used hot water bottles with warm water or one or two Fleet's enemas. I will discuss this in more detail in the chapter on labor.

12. *Oral and rectal thermometers.* The mother needs to have her temperature taken orally during labor and the days following the labor. The baby may need to have the temperature taken rectally.

13. *Isopropyl alcohol.* To apply to the stump of the baby's umbilical cord after each diaper change.

14. *Candles or lanterns.* Nearly everyone likes soft lights during the labor and delivery.

15. *Bowl for placenta.* This bowl should be medium size.

16. *Bendable straws* for drinking while lying down.

17. *Lip balm and hair ties.*

18. *Miso soup and good nourishing foods* to have while laboring and after the birth.

19. *Baby clothes.* Such items as baby gowns with draw strings, undershirts, diapers, receiving blankets.

20. *Adequate heat source in the house* (at least 70° F).

21. *Sterilized sheets.* Two sets of sheets for making up the bed as described above with the drop cloth. Women have told me that they have sterilized their sheets by going to a commercial laundromat. They put the sheets in an unused plastic bag and sealed the bag with tape. This is to be done at least two weeks before the due date.

22. *Honey or maple syrup.* When the laboring woman needs a shot of quick energy, honey or maple syrup can be put in some water or juice and drunk right down.

23. *Herb teas* as desired. Check with your midwife to see what herbs she uses.

24. *Toilet paper.*

25. *Baby cosmetics.* Cornstarch or baby powder; Weleda baby oil; calendula ointment or cream.

26. *Large paper bags* for disposing things.

27. *Emergency Childbirth* by Dr. Gregory White.

28. *Food and a place to sleep to offer attendants.*

29. *Phone numbers of attendants in a handy place.* I tell people to tape the numbers to the phone.

30. *Plastic squirt bottle.* This could be an empty shampoo bottle, or you can buy them at the store. This bottle is to be filled with warm water and kept by the toilet, so that when the mother urinates after the birth she can squirt this on herself while she is urinating. It stops the stinging.

31. *Six pairs of sterile gloves* for the birth attendant. Make sure that they are the right size for her hand.

32. *Plastic dishpan.* This is for a footbath, which is used for rinsing the feet when the mother gets in and out of the tank. I have made the concentration of one-half betadine to one-half water.

33. *Aquarium fishnet* (or fondly referred to as a pooper-scooper). A medium-sized net is best and is used for scooping out any vomit, blood clots, or pieces of feces that may get into the tank.

34. *Pool thermometer.* For making sure that the tank is at the proper temperature.

35. *Children's pool rafts or rings.* For leaning against while in labor.

Pregnancy is such a beautiful time in a woman's life—despite the nausea, the backaches, and the headaches, and the swinging hormones, and the feelings of being a beached whale toward the end of the pregnancy. I feel sad when I hear some women complain about being pregnant throughout their pregnancy. It is as if they forget to look on the bright side and to see what a blessing it is to have life growing inside of them. I felt so close to God when I was pregnant. For me, it is a miracle to feel the kicks and movements of life. It is fascinating to watch the belly grow bigger as the baby grows inside. I feel privileged to be a woman because I can carry life inside and give birth to life. This is why I always tell my couples to enjoy their pregnancy. The nine months really do go by very fast. If this is her first baby, a woman should relish her time alone, while still feeling the movements of another life within her. What could be more beautiful, I tell them, than feeling life in you, to have that little someone be part of your flesh and blood? Going through the different phases of pregnancy can be a fulfilling and empowering experience in womanhood.

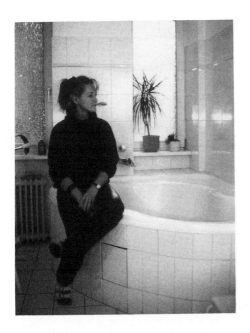

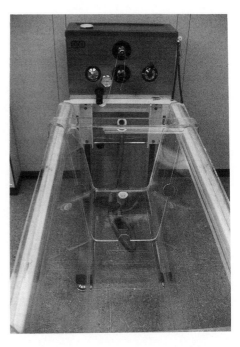

Maureen Amonis, in her clinic in Berlin, Germany. Photograph by the author

Tub at a birth clinic in Oodense, Berlin. Photograph by the author

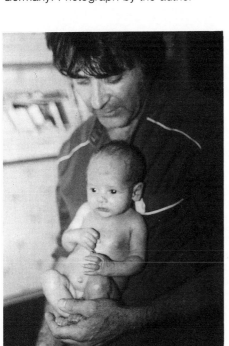

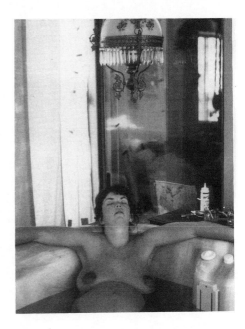

Igor Charkowsky with a baby born in water. Photograph by the author

Sleeping in the tub in between contractions. Photograph by Robert Kraus

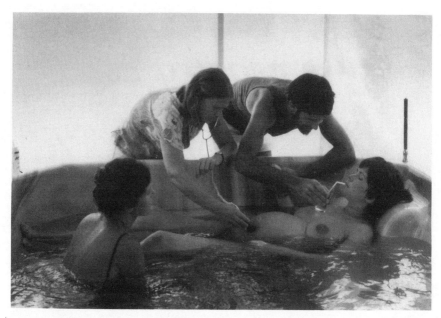

Water allows laboring mothers to lie comfortably on their backs. Photograph by Robert Kraus

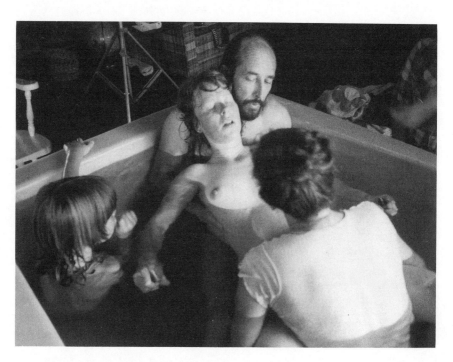

With help from her family and the midwife, a mother relaxes while in labor. Photograph by Robert Kraus

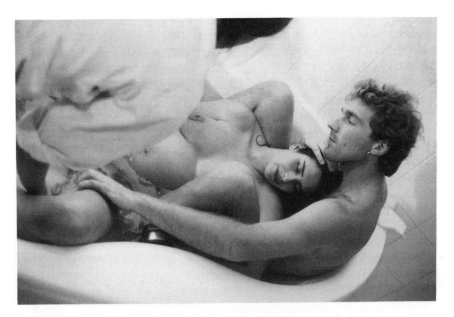

Father supporting laboring mother at a birth clinic in Berlin, Germany. Photograph by the author

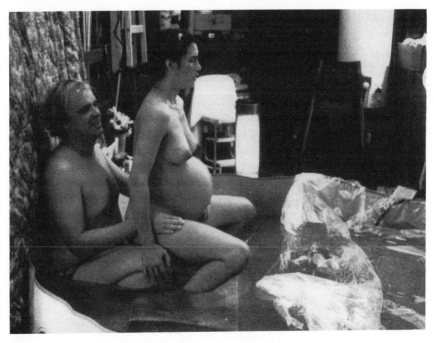

The partner can be used as a birthing chair to work with gravity. Photograph by Portia Blau

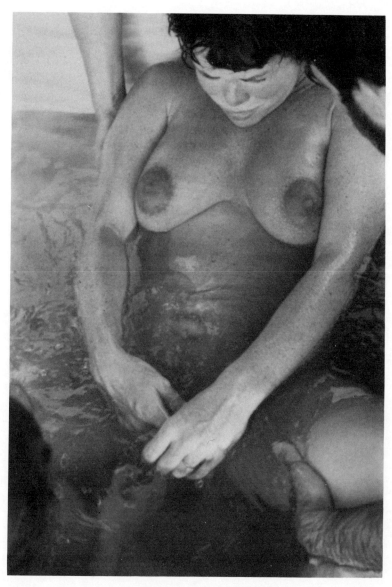

Put your chin down into your chest, roll your shoulders forward and
push down and out! Photograph by Robert Kraus

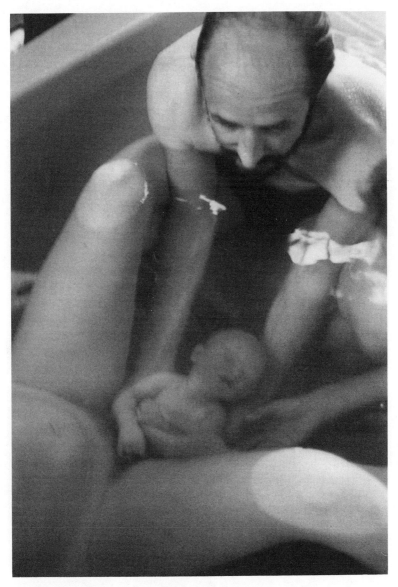

Catching the baby is a wonderful experience for the father. Photograph by Irene Tefft

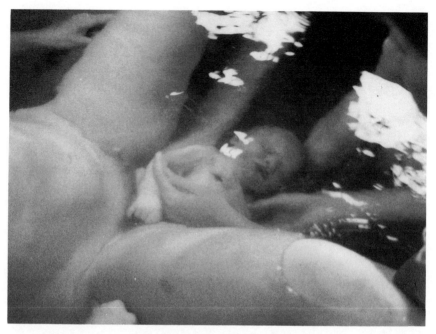

The baby's body may slowly emerge to the chest. Photograph by Robert Kraus

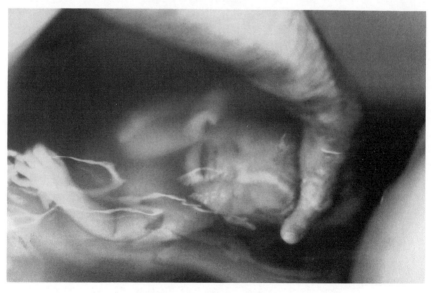

Many infants born in water appear to be asleep; they do not seem to know that they have been born. Photograph by Robert Kraus

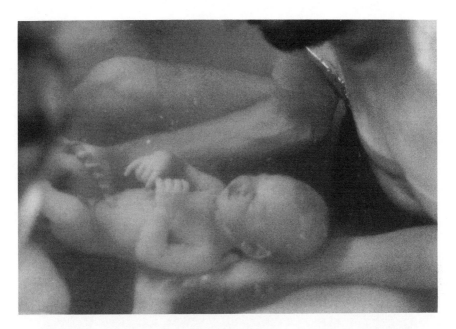

The baby after a few seconds underwater. Photograph by Robert Kraus

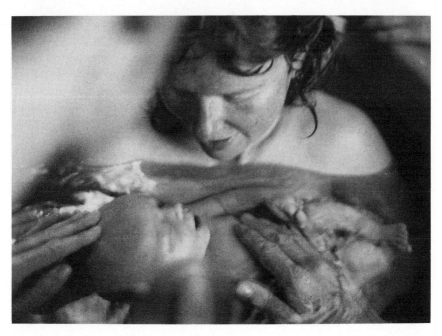

After being brought to the surface, the baby is calm and appears to be sleeping. Photograph by Robert Kraus

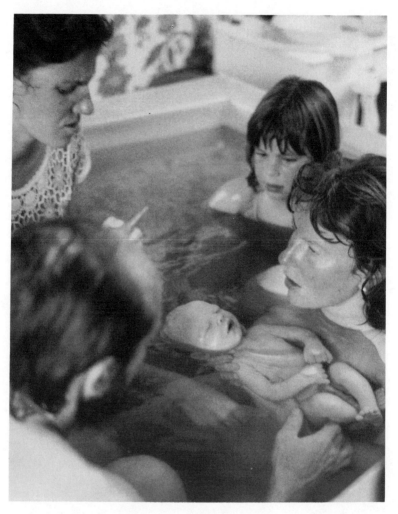

Leaving the baby's body in the water and the face out, so that he can
breathe. Photograph by Robert Kraus

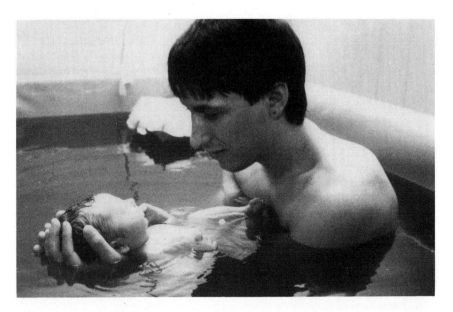

The babies seem to love the water. Photograph by the author

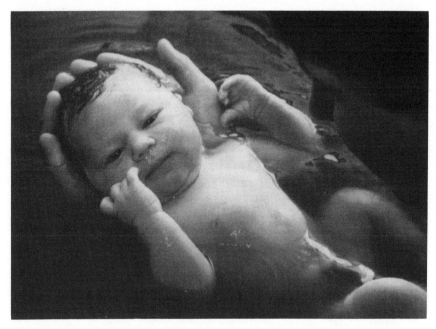

The newborn is content and alert after being brought to the surface. Photograph by the author

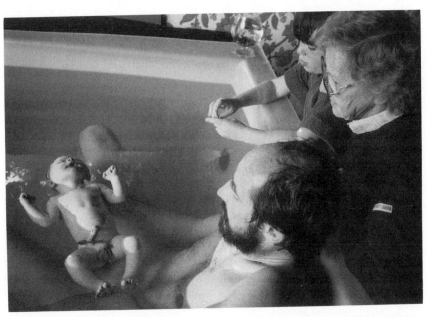

Family bonding time can begin right after birth. Photograph by Robert Kraus

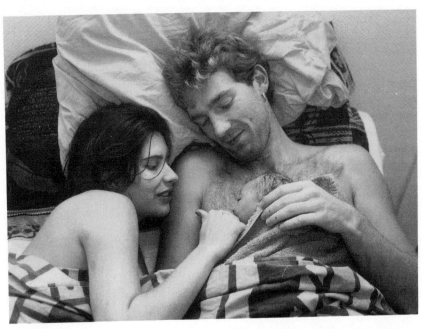

Mother, father, and newborn snuggling in Berlin, Germany. Photograph by the author

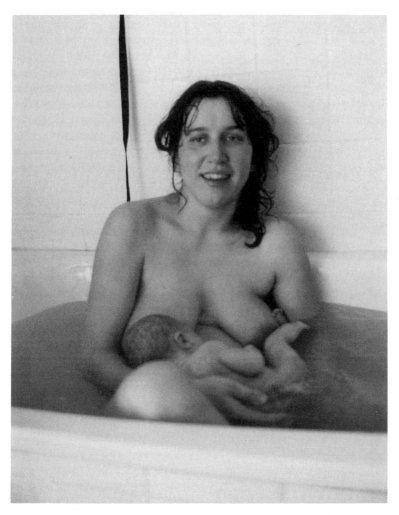

A healthy mother and baby minutes after birth in Berlin, Germany.
Photograph by the author

5

TANKS

Several different types of tanks have been used for underwater births. Igor Charkowsky's plexiglass tank is wonderful for the visual aspects of the water birth. Charkowsky has his own tank, which is set up at the home of the pregnant mother. The tank is also used for swimming instructions for the infants and toddlers. It is ideal for making movies and taking photographs. Yet I question how the water would be kept at a constant temperature. One would have to have an apartment-complex-size water heater to maintain a temperature of 100° F (38° C) for any length of time.

During my pregnancy, I rented a fiberglass spa that had jacuzzi jets as part of the tank. It was set up in my living room about three weeks in advance. Having an enormous amount of low back pain in my ninth month, I often sat in the tank with the jets on the small of my back. It gave great relief; I remember thinking that every woman should have this luxury. The jets are of value while laboring for two reasons: It is a relief to have the jets massaging your back while in labor; and the jets help to keep the water circulating. In most tanks, when the jets are on, the filtering system is on as well as the heating system. This is not true with all tanks. One should investigate these matters carefully when buying or renting.

The spas can come in various sizes, shapes, and materials. Two or more people should be able to fit comfortably in the tank. They usually have a flat bench to sit on or contoured seats that allow various positions. I worked with a woman who was over six feet tall and had a jacuzzi spa that she could lie down in. Remember to take into consideration your needs, finances, the amount of space the tank will take, the weight of the filled tank, and the strength of the house supports. If all this is feasible, then a jacuzzi spa would be a wonderful investment. Many people reuse the spa to teach the baby to swim in it.

Inflatable hot tubs have recently come on the market. They are made of strong vinyl and appear to be strong enough to lean up against for support while in labor. The tank has plenty of room for women to move around and get into different positions. Depending on the size, two to three people could comfortably fit into them. I haven't worked with these tanks, but have heard mixed reports from people who have used them. Some say the sides are not strong enough to support a mother leaning on them, but others say they are fine.

On the opposite end of the economic scale is the child's wading pool which can be purchased at any toy store. The pools can range anywhere from 5 feet to 9 feet in diameter and from 18 inches to 25 inches deep. Waterbed heaters can be placed underneath the tank. Usually, about two to three heaters are necessary. With the thermostat control on the heaters, the water temperature can be regulated. A space blanket can be kept under the heaters with the reflective side up. This helps the heat go up into the tank, and at the same time the floor is protected. It may be wise to put a blanket underneath the space blanket for added protection and padding. As for having something to lean up against, this tank functions minimally. One cannot lean up against the sides, or water will spill out. One couple set their wading pool in the garage, both for the weight and to be able to put the tank up against the wall so that when someone leaned against the side, there would be support and a lot of water would not come spilling out. Plastic should be put on the floor around the base of the tank so that the carpet or floors do not get all wet.

In California, in the early 1980s, a few women gave birth in unused horse troughs that were freshly painted. I have never worked with these tanks. In an interview, the woman stated that they found them to be roomy enough to move around in and strong enough to support anyone who leaned against them. As in Charkowsky's plexiglass tank, however, there is no way to keep this tank at a constant temperature. The people who used the horse troughs also told me that they connected the hose to the hot water heater and brought the water in that way. Most warned me about draining the hot water heater, because there is usually sediment on the bottom of the hot water tank and this can get into the horse trough. It is important to have the birthing area as clean as possible.

In some cases, when the hot water runs out some have had to shuffle pans of hot water that have been heated on the stove. If this is the case, then an extra pair of hands should be invited to the birth and assigned to that task.

Bathtubs are not the greatest tubs for laboring in, because they do not give the mother enough freedom of movement. She basically has to stay in a semisitting position if she wants to birth in water. This does not allow for freedom of expression while laboring or giving birth. Unless one has a sunken Japanese bath or a large European-size bath, it may be hard to squat in a conventional American-size bath, which seems to be built for birds. Maintaining the temperature of the water, as in some of the other tanks, is also tricky. Since the water is so shallow, it cools off a lot more quickly. This problem could also be alleviated with someone keeping the kettle on the stove to add water to the tub.

I would not feel comfortable assisting a mother to labor or birth her baby in a wooden hot tub, mainly because wood harbors bacteria. If the tank has been used previous to the labor, it may have bacteria in the wood that you wouldn't want at a birth, especially if people other than your own family have been in it. Staph is nasty and tough and loves to hang out in such places. The wood is often treated or sealed with toxic chemicals that may be fine for adults, but would you want your new-born exposed to it?

Sea salt should be added to the water. Dr. Odent does not add salt, and Igor Charkowsky does. I think that one must follow one's own intuition on this matter. Here are the reasons why I like salt: Salt is a natural antibacterial substance. Since the mother may defecate in the tank, precautions need to be taken to ensure the health of mother and baby. Salt also adds buoyancy to the water, which gives even more freedom of movement while laboring. Salt also helps to maintain the water temperature. Salt is one of the main constituents of amniotic fluid. When the baby is born, he tastes the water. Environmental factors are theorized to stimulate breathing in the newborn. When the newborn tastes the salt, it will be the same as the taste he has been familiar with for nine months.

An equation has been used to determine the amount of salt needed for your own personal tank. This equation will mock the salinity of amniotic fluid:

0.0003 pound of salt × cubic inches of water in the tank = amount of salt to put in water.

There are 231 cubic inches in one gallon of water. If we can figure out how many gallons of water the tank holds, then arriving at the answer will be easy. The water should taste like sea water. Charkowsky believes that sea water is the best medium for birth.

In the early days of attending water births, some people found it difficult to obtain a suitable tank to give birth in. Either they were too expensive, the time and the skills were lacking to build a tank, or wading pools sometimes were not appropriate. The first two families with whom I worked built their own tanks. Then I worked with families who didn't have the time to build them and used various kinds of tanks.

When Jeff René built his tank for the birth of his child, I was very impressed with the simplicity and efficiency of the tank. Both his daughters were eventually born in the same type of tank. Jeff has been building and renting out his tanks since 1984; over 120 couples have used them. I can't sing their praises enough. I asked Jeff to describe how to build the tanks. Here is how he does it!

A BIRTH TUB ODYSSEY

What I decided to do was to construct a modular frame that could be disassembled into four walls and a bottom panel. These were put together with 2 × 4 fir, ½ inch A/C plywood, plastic moisture barriers, and standard fiberglass insulation. Once the frame is assembled, a pad and insulation are set in the bottom. Waterbed heating elements that plug into standard household current are taped to the inside walls, which are lined with a fitted vinyl (potable water designated) liner. A 6 mil plastic sheet is placed over the tank after it is prepared and filled in order to keep out dust and bugs and to hold in moisture. Finally, a thermal barrier, such as a blanket, is put over the top to hold in heat.

You should be able to buy all frame materials, heaters, liner, and all your miscellaneous equipment for $300 to $350 new, plus your labor. A tub system can be used over and over, simply replacing a plywood panel, heater, or liner when worn or suspect. The average cost for the equipment wear, cleaners, disinfectant, and material has averaged $60 to $80 for a birth.

TUB FRAME CONSTRUCTION

Materials:

Three 4 × 8 ft sheets of A/C ½" plywood

Eight 8 ft 2 × 4 KD fir

20 ft R-19 fiberglass insulation 15" wide

One 10 × 20 ft sheet 6 mil polyethylene clear plastic tarp

1¼" and 1⅝" sheetrock screws (100 of each will be enough)

12d. framing and 12d. finish nails (32 of each)

Tube of latex caulking

½ gal water-based polyurethane

Small can of wood putty

Diagram A

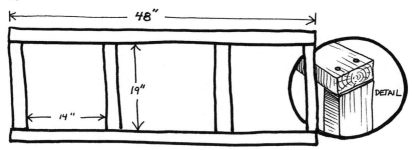

Diagram by Jeff Cox

Tools:

Circular saw
Drill
Hammer
Nail set
Countersink
Screwdriver gun
Carpenter square
Caulking gun
Plywood blade for saw
Staple gun (light duty Arrow JT-21 is perfect)
Orbital sander with 100 grit paper

Begin with the 2 × 4's, and cut eight 48" 2 × 4's, selecting the straightest for the top and bottom rails; then cut sixteen 19" 2 × 4's for the uprights in the frame. Mark these with the carpenter's square to get nice 90 degree cuts. Per Diagram A, nail the frames together with two finish nails on the top and two framing nails on the bottom on each upright. Set the finish nails ¼" into the top rail with a nail set and fill the holes with wood putty. Set your frames aside.

Next cut the plywood per Diagram B.

Take the four inner wall plywood panels and countersink per Diagram C on the clean side of the plywood. These will set the screw heads into the wood without splintering the plywood, leaving flat sides. The side panels could be nailed on, but the screws enable you to easily replace any panel that may be damaged. I don't actually drill a hole through the plywood: instead, I leave a nub of drill so it doesn't wander, and countersink only to create a beveled cut to seat the screws and avoid splin-

Diagram B

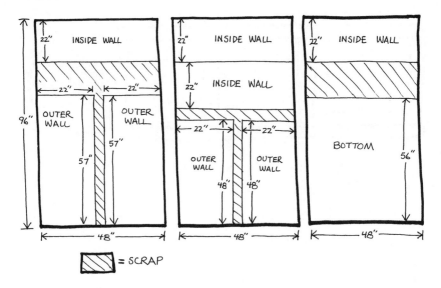

Diagram by Jeff Cox

tering. A screwdriver gun will drive the screw and seat the screw head without a hole being drilled.

Now let's assemble the walls (Diagram C). Lay one of the 2 × 4 frames on a table with the bottom toward you and use your caulking gun to put an ⅛" bead of caulk down the middle of all the outer 2 × 4's: top, bottom, and ends. Lay some of your 6 mil plastic moisture barrier over the frame and staple into place, and cut the plastic ¼" back from the edge with a knife or razor blade. Cover one side on all four frames. Lay another ⅛" bead of caulking over the plastic following the bead that you put on under the plastic, lay the plywood over the frame and plastic, and flush up at the top edge and corners. Drive the five 1¼" screws on the top edge first; then, if you have cut the plywood accurately, adjusting the frame to the plywood will produce a squared wall section. Just give any protruding frame end a whack with your hammer in order to square it and complete driving 1¼" screws in your countersinks. Do the same on all four wall sections.

Turn the frames over, cut your insulation into 20" lengths with scissors, push the insulation into the frames with the paper or foil side toward you, and staple every 4" all around. With a knife or razor blade, cut the excess paper to ¾" from the outside edge. Run another ⅛" bead of caulk right along the cut, which is in the middle of the 2 × 4, and staple your 6 mil plastic moisture barrier over the frame and insulation, again trimming to ¼" back from the outer edge.

Diagram C

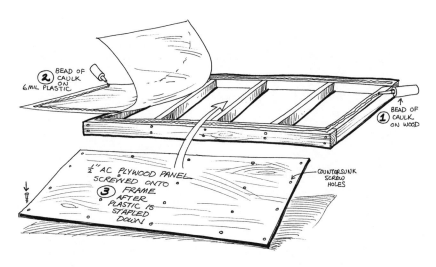

Diagram by Jeff Cox

Diagram D

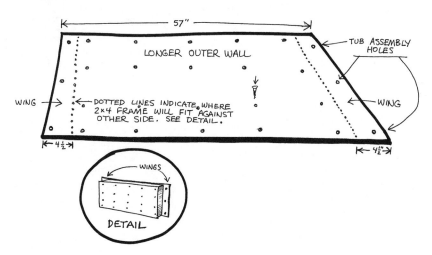

Diagram by Jeff Cox

Now we put on the four plywood outer panels. Notice that two of the outer walls are 57" and two are 48". Drill your countersinks on the smaller outer walls exactly as you did on the first four, but, on the two larger outer walls, the countersinks should be drilled as shown in Diagram D.

Diagram E

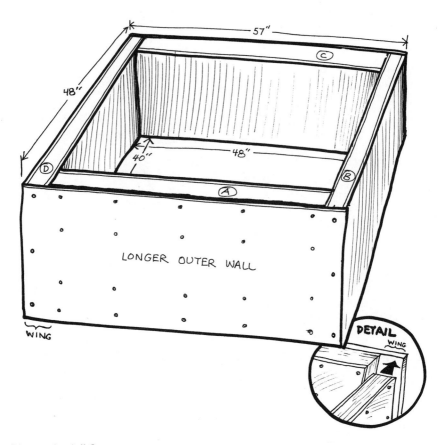

Diagram by Jeff Cox

Assemble the short outer panels as you did the inners. Run ⅛" bead of caulking, flush top and ends, fasten with 1¼" screws, but let the plywood find the best square position on the frame first. The frame is less adjustable now. Fill all the countersinks with 1¼" screws and drive them.

On the larger outer panels, pencil mark 4½" back from the ends along both top and bottom, lay on the bead of caulk, then line these marks up with ends of the frame both top and bottom, screw top countersinks first, then drive a 1¼" screw in each countersink except the three drilled tub assembly holes at the ends. We now have two rectangular insulated walls and two similar walls with 4½" extended wings.

We need to drill a 1⅛" wiring hole 9" up from the bottom centered at 7" in from the end on the outer panel of one wing wall, and 2¼" in from

Diagram F

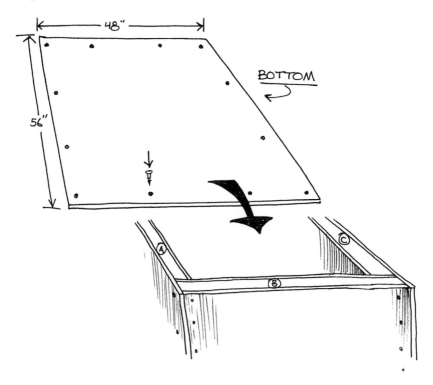

Diagram by Jeff Cox

the end on the inner panel, to pass heating element wires and thermo-static sensor through the wall.

We are ready to assemble the four walls, building the frame upside down. Lay the walls on the top edge, with the wing walls opposite each other (Diagram E). You will be looking at the edge with the framing nail heads facing you.

Butt the rectangular walls into the corners created by the wings all around, keeping them flush with each other across the top. While holding the walls snugly together, drive 1⅝" screws through the three predrilled countersink holes in the wings. The four walls are now assembled and should be marked A, B, C, D, so that they may be easily assembled and disassembled and all screw holes will align each time. Use permanent ink.

The last building task is to lay the bottom plywood panel over the frame with the good side away from you. (On all other panels we drilled the countersink holes in the better side plywood surface; on the bottom the countersinks will be in the rougher side.) You should have the bottom edge of the outer wall plywood showing equally all around. Countersink

and drill twelve holes in the plywood per Diagram F. Drive twelve 1⅝"
screws through these holes to secure the bottom. You now have the tub
frame constructed and marked. To disassemble: remove the twelve bottom screws and set the bottom aside; remove the three outer screws
from each wing wall (twelve in all), and put your twenty-four 1⅝" assembly screws in a container.

It will only take you ten minutes with a screwdriver gun to assemble
or disassemble the five frame components.

You should now look over the edges of the plywood and 2 × 4's and
fill any gaps with wood putty. Take your orbital sander and round all your
edges of each panel, especially the bottom, to keep them from splintering; sand all faces and countersink areas, the wire holes—reassemble
the walls and bottom, and turn the tub frame over. I like to give a little
extra attention to the top outer edge in its assembled position and to the
area where the wall sections come together. Disassemble the frame by
turning it over and removing the twenty-four screws.

The last task with the frame is to seal with two coats of water-based
polyurethane and allow them proper drying time.

HEATERS

The simplest way to maintain water temperature is with waterbed-style
heating pads. They are efficient, obtainable anywhere, run on standard
current, and come in a variety of styles. Each heating pad comes with
a thermostatic control unit and sensor.

I incorporate two heating pads and controls in this design. While only
one heating pad is necessary to maintain water temperature, the second
is very useful: as a backup if one should break; and to bring the water
up to temperature initially. During a long labor or birth, air drafting can
knock down the water temperature.

I have used all kinds of these heaters and find that 10"–12" wide pads,
30"–36" long are the best size. Don't buy a heating pad that is too wide
for the water depth or too long for the tub frame; leave clear space at
both ends. I use duo-therm heaters because the heating pad doesn't
delaminate with taping and untaping the pad to and from the tub wall.

The heater pads mount to the walls of the tub with masking tape (don't
use thick glue tapes like duct tape), which is only meant to hold the
heater pad in place until the weight of the water is added. Mount the
heaters 2" up from the bottom of the tub, so that the electrical cords take
a gentle bend into the wiring hole, and secure the wire with masking
tape. It is important to mount the heating pad flat, without creases or air
spaces that can cause overheating in that part of the element. I don't
think it is safe to place the heater pads on the bottom of the frame because they would take more abuse from being stepped on and because

a leaking liner could place your heating pad directly in contact with water.

I handle each of the control units differently. On the first control I gently uncoil the sensor line and pass it through the wiring hole from the outside in under the element wires. Mount the control switch, with the screws provided, somewhere above and to the side of the wire hole far enough so that the wire and sensor take a gentle bend. Bend the sensor line down toward the corner or the frame with rounded bends, and locate the sensor bulb on the bottom panel 1" from and along the wall. Tape the sensor line so that it sits flat on the wall and the sensor bulb flat to the bottom, with masking tape. If you put several layers of tape over the bulb, you can extend the range of the control beyond 100° F simply by insulating the sensor bulb with tape. Shake the element wires so that you know which heater is your controlled heating pad, and plug the pad wire into the control, coiling the excess wire up out of the way. You will use this control dial to maintain the temperature of your water.

On the second control unit, I uncoil the sensor tube and wrap the tube around the control unit, with the sensor sticking up; turn the temperature dial to the highest position; and wrap the unit with masking tape. This is your backup heater; as long as the air temperature is less than 100° F, your heating pad will be on when the unit is plugged in. The backup heater is generally used to bring the water temperature up, or to maintain the water temperature while using the tub before and during the birth. Other than that it is left unplugged unless the other pad should malfunction. Never plug the heaters in and turn them on if there is no water in the tank or the water is not completely covering them. Also, never leave them plugged into power while draining the tub. Use a spa thermometer or pool thermometer to monitor water temperature.

BOTTOM INSULATION/PAD

Before adding the liner to the frame, it is good to add a bottom pad cut or folded 2" to 3" from the side walls all around. This would be a pad 34" to 36" wide and 42" to 44" long. A ¾" insulite camping pad or 1" foam pad work well, but I generally fold a blanket into the bottom of the frame leaving the 2" to 3" space all around. The pad creates a depression which helps the collection of liquids used in cleaning the liner.

THE LINER

To line the frame, I selected a 30 mil vinyl, potable water designated liner. These are generally used to line drinking water storage tanks and are fabricated to specification. A 25 mil vinyl is acceptable but doesn't have the same wear characteristics as the 30 mil vinyl. This material is very durable, but it will cut easily if placed on a sharp object.

Any vinyl swimming pool manufacturer or vinyl fabricator can make your liner. Order a 40" wide by 48" long by 22" deep liner. They will ask you how much edge you want at the top, and 2" top edge works fine. When ordering a broader top edge, I've found that the fit has been less precise. A good fit to the frame is important.

Make sure that nothing sharp is embedded in your bottom pad, that no splinters are in the frame wood, and that any sharp moulding points in the heat pads are masked with tape. Bring the four corners up to the top corners of the frame and staple at the corners only, using a light-duty staple gun (like the Arrow JT-21.) As you are filling the tub, then you will want to add more staples to the sides to keep the liner in place. Spread the liner to fit the frame with your hands. You want to make sure that the liner fits the corners well but, more importantly, that it sits flat over the heater pads, without creases or air spaces.

After trying other ways of fastening, I've come to the conclusion that staples are simplest and best. The tub is now complete.

EQUIPMENT TO COMPLETE THE SYSTEM

Top moisture barrier. Use the piece of 6 mil clear plastic for putting over the tub to prevent the heat from escaping. Do not cover the tub when it is occupied.

Hoses. A garden or drinking water hose is used for filling and draining the tub. You may have noticed that no drains are incorporated in the liner. Siphoning with a hose to a lower point than the tub bottom, or using a waterbed or aquarium siphon that attaches to a sink or tub faucet is entirely adequate.

Filtering Equipment. I like clear filter bodies for 9¾" standard, full-flow filters. I use Ametek filter bodies because they are inexpensive and available all over the United States.

OTHER CONSIDERATIONS

Before assembling your tub, consider the structural site. All modern construction will hold the tub and water weight easily. In older wood frame construction that may have insect or water damage, or in the case of large span floors, place the tub closer to an outside sustaining wall, over a wall or support below, or, as in a "crawl space" situation, tack a 4 × 4 support post under the center of the tub site, to limit floor deflection. It's more of a worry than a problem. I've never seen structural damage from the tub weight. A filled tub will weigh approximately ¾ ton or 1,500 pounds.

Use tincture of green soap to scrub the liner or a betadine solution before filling and after draining the tub.

Enjoy your tub and happy birthing!

Author's addition: An important point to consider is the location of the toilet. Because laboring mothers often need to use the facility while in labor, it can be difficult if the toilet is on the second floor and the tub is located on the first floor. Long distances to the toilet can be tiring after a while. Another point to consider is that a foam mat or some sort of bed is placed right next to the tub, in case there is an emergency and the mother needs to get out of the tub quickly. The bed should not be in the next room.

6

===

LABORING IN WATER

Dr. Michel Odent emphasizes that it was never intended that the laboring mothers he has worked with at the Centre Hospitalier General in Pithiviers should give birth in water. Actually, the women who come to the hospital are encouraged to labor in any way they want, using their intuition. To encourage women to use intuition in laboring, a tank of warm water is available. Dr. Odent states that immersion in warm water helps mothers lose their inhibitions while laboring. Therefore, when the laboring mothers come to the second stage, the pushing stage, they do not want to get out of the tank. The babies are born peacefully into the water, even though this was not the intent.

Using water while pregnant and in labor assists women in many ways. The weight of the baby on the lower back during the last few days of pregnancy can at times be unbearable. During my pregnancy, I had been suffering from low back pain for two days, and so I began to use a tank of water that had been set up in the corner of my living room for my forthcoming water birth. I used the warm water and the water jets to ease the discomfort. It made me buoyant, which helped me to relax. The weight of the baby immediately lifted, and the discomfort was gone. I can't imagine going through those last few days without it. As my back pain became more intense and more difficult to alleviate, I thought I had thrown my back out, but I started checking myself vaginally and found that I was dilating. Labor had begun.

I have had a lifelong affinity for water, and now that I was in labor, I was glad to have the tank near me. I loved the soothing, sensual feeling of the warm water. The contractions felt less intense, as I was able to rock my body back and forth and get into positions I knew would help the progress of the birth and ease the discomfort. I would get out of the tank when I felt the necessity to work with gravity, and I would get back in when the contractions became too fierce, when I felt overwhelmed by their intensity. As soon as my legs slid under the warm liquid, I could feel my whole body relax. While in the tank, I thought hollow: be a hollow tube; let the baby come through; be open to dilation. The water helped calm me, encouraging me to collect myself and remind myself that women have been giving birth since the beginning of time.

Shortly before midnight, I was dilated 1 centimeter. As the night progressed, I dilated a centimeter an hour. At 5:30 A.M., Nathaniel's amniotic sac broke. I was 5 centimeters. I happened to be out of the tank when I had an intense contraction. All I could do was to get back into the tank. Immediately, I felt the urge to push. There was no stopping me. I could not hold back. I was checked and found to be completely dilated. A few pushes later, Nathaniel was born. From the time the bag of waters broke at 5 centimeters until the birth, one half hour had gone by—an incredibly fast time for a first-time mother. The total time of my labor and delivery was six hours. I used many resources from my midwife's bag of tricks in this labor, but I believe that being in the water during the first stage played a major role in its rapid completion.

I cannot imagine being without water during labor. Some practitioners discourage the use of water until the woman is in hard labor. No one could have kept me out. The water helped me relax, enabling me to call upon my instincts to do whatever was needed to birth this baby in the way I needed. This personal experience with water and labor supported what I had already discovered in attending water births—that water has a positive and beneficial effect available to the majority of pregnant women. As a midwife I saw it; as a mother, I experienced it.

GETTING READY FOR LABOR AND THE FIRST STAGE

For many women, the last few weeks of pregnancy can be filled with mixed emotions. Many women enjoy being pregnant so much that the thought of giving up the "oneness" that bonds mother and baby can be saddening. On the other hand, many women look forward to being able to hold their baby in their arms. The last few weeks of pregnancy can also be times of discomfort; the baby is putting pressure on the lower back and against the bladder, the hands and feet of the mother may be swelling, and moving is becoming awkward. What is worse, everyone is calling and asking if the baby has arrived yet. Every day is filled with the anticipation of the little one's arrival, with searching for every little sign that labor may be starting. New parents are not quite sure what to expect, even though they may have read all the literature and attended the best childbirth classes. The best thing one can do is relax and enjoy the last few days of having the baby moving around inside. The nine months of pregnancy fly by so quickly that only a few months after the baby is born, pregnancy feels as if it had been a dream. Be in close contact with your midwife or doctor and your body will know the rest. Your body will know what to do and will give you all the signals.

A few days before the woman goes into labor, hormonal shifts start occurring. Women say that they feel "different." Some women become very elated, as if someone slipped them a drug; others become very moody. Many women can feel the extreme mood changes, while others are frantically cleaning the house enjoying the nesting instinct.

PRELIMINARY LABOR OR FALSE LABOR

So-called false labor can at times appear to be true labor. The mother starts feeling contractions, but after a few hours, the intensity just fades away. I have never liked the term *false labor*. It has such a negative sound, leaving the mother feeling inadequate and disappointed. Instead, I prefer to describe the situation as preliminary labor. I almost always find that these contractions accomplish something, even though they eventually stop. These shortlived contractions help lower the baby further into the birth canal and can assist in the dilation and effacement of the cervix. Thus, even though it may be a small amount, something is accomplished.

Women may become overly excited at the thought of seeing their baby. I caution them that this surge of adrenalin may also prevent them from sleeping. This inability to sleep can be mistaken for a sign of labor. Sleep is one of the most important things that the mother and father can do to prepare for labor. Sleep helps to give the mind and body energy to work the hardest it has probably ever worked. Severe complications may arise from lack of it. The father also needs his sleep, for without it he may not be able to function as a good support person, to make informed decisions, or to catch his baby. I cannot emphasize enough the importance of sleeping or at the very least resting before going into true labor. The mother's body needs lots of rest and strength to work efficiently to get the baby out. Without sufficient rest, the mother's body may become exhausted and unable to work properly. The baby in turn may become stressed. With a tired mother and stressed baby, it may be necessary to go to the hospital. So please sleep!

I can remember attending a mother who was so sure she was in labor that she had been up for several hours in the middle of the night. After arriving at her home and spending time with her, I realized that it was not true labor. Encouraging her to get in a warm shower was the best thing to do. The warm water relaxed her. Her husband brought her a few sips of wine and a cup of camomile tea. The mild contractions stopped completely, and she was off to sleep. If she had been in true labor, her relaxed body would have gone into harder labor and sleep would have been nearly impossible.

TRUE LABOR

When the water breaks and increasingly strong and regular contractions begin within a few hours, true labor is most likely underway and the mother can use the water tank as she sees fit. However, the onset of labor does not always begin with the breaking of the waters.

Most midwives want to be alerted as soon as possible that labor has begun. They will want to know if the water has broken, what color the water is, and how far apart the contractions are. Timing the contractions helps let the practitioner know how far along the labor is. If you have a watch with a second hand, finding out how far apart they are is very easy. Count the time from the beginning of the first contraction to the beginning of the next contraction. The "duration" of a contraction is a different measurement—it is counted from its beginning to its end.

These are a few of the other signs of the onset of true labor:

1. Contractions that get progressively stronger and progressively longer, and come closer together.

2. A feeling similar to menstrual cramps, and a little bit of blood when she wipes herself after urinating. This is often due to the blood vessels breaking in the cervix as the contractions lower the baby further into the pelvis, thinning (effacing) and dilating the cervix.

3. The continual leaking of amniotic fluid, its presence having been confirmed by nitrazine paper. (If you have just made love, semen can also show positive on nitrazine paper. Wait for an hour or two, then check.)

4. Strong contractions that keep the woman awake. It is impossible to sleep.

During the first stage of labor, the cervix effaces and dilates from 0 to 10 centimeters. Along with the cervical dilation, the baby is decending into the birth canal. At 10 centimeters, the cervix is completely dilated and the mother enters the second stage, when she pushes the baby out.

The effacement or thinning of the cervix is accomplished by both the internal and external opening (os) of the cervix. (The cervix is the opening of the uterus.) During a contraction, the top segment of the uterus contracts and pulls up on the lower segment of the uterus (the cervix), thinning the cervix out. Meanwhile, the baby's head is descending

Figure 2
The Various Stations during the Descent of the Baby's Head through the Pelvis

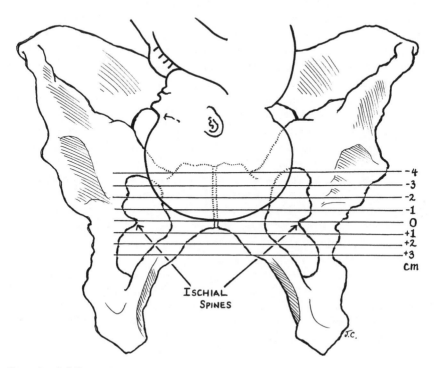

-4
-3
-2
-1
0
+1
+2
+3
cm

ISCHIAL
SPINES

J.C.

Figure by Jeff Cox

lower into the pelvis and is assisting in the effacement as well as the dilation of the cervix.

The ischial spines are two promontory bones that are part of the mother's pelvis. They are said to be 0 (zero) station when the baby's head is "engaged." The descent of the baby's head into the mother's pelvis is called the stations. It is possible that other parts of the baby's body may be presenting (going down first), such as the buttocks or feet. To eliminate confusion, I speak in terms of the head as the presenting part. The stations are measured in terms of centimeters, that is, −5 station resting high above the ischial spines, −4 station 1 centimeter closer to the ischial spines, −3, −2, −1, and 0 stations. Below the ischial spines, the baby is lowering her head into the mother's pelvis. At +4 station or +5 station, the baby is at the opening of the vagina (vaginal orifice.)

With a first-time mom (a primipara), the engagement of the baby's head with the ischial spines occurs approximately two weeks before the due date. A multipara (a mother who has given birth to more than one child) may go into labor with the head of the baby not yet engaged—and it may not engage until a few hours into labor.

During the early part of the first stage (from 0 to 4 centimeters), the baby's head descends into the proper position and the cervix dilates and effaces. At first, contractions may come every half hour and gradually increase in duration and intensity. They may be more "bearable" in this early period. When I arrive at the home of the laboring mother and I find her laughing and joking, this clues me into how far along she is in her labor. At this point she may feel that the labor is easy. Getting in the tank can help her relax and dilate faster if she finds the water inviting. With most first-time mothers, labor is longer, and more work needs to be done to get the baby out. Hanging out in the tub for long periods of time (a half hour to an hour) may be self-defeating. It is good to get up and move, and work with gravity to help the baby get further down into the birth canal. The laboring mother can get back into the tank after a time when the contractions have picked up a bit more. If the contractions start slowing down again while in the water, it is best to get out and work with gravity.

I usually encourage women to sleep during the very early stages of labor so that they have plenty of strength and energy when the hard work needs to be done. When sleep is no longer possible, I advise them to go about their everyday affairs or go for walks. If sitting or lying down feels more comfortable, I encourage them to change positions frequently. If the woman is lying on her side for a long period of time, I encourage her to roll over to the other side or sit up. Staying in one position does not facilitate the baby's ability to go further down into the birth canal. Laboring mothers may find a comfortable position, one where they can "stand" the contractions. Moving around, getting into the upright position, walking, and squatting positions work with the force of gravity to bring the baby lower into the birth canal. Comfortable positions may just postpone the inevitable—good, hard-working contractions that are necessary to get the baby out that often hurt. In the pushing stage (second stage), working with gravity is also a necessity, because it helps the body work in so many different ways to push the baby out.

Freedom of movement while in labor has become lost in the "civilized" world. Women are made to lie in bed, hooked up to machines, unable to move around. One of nature's most important gifts to aiding labor—gravity—has been forgotten. Women have used the squatting and upright positions while in labor since time began. While the baby is being born, his head must go through a spiraling motion in the pelvis. Birth is asymmetrical. In order for the labor to progress well, to help the baby

Figure 3
Ways of Laboring and Birthing among Primitive People

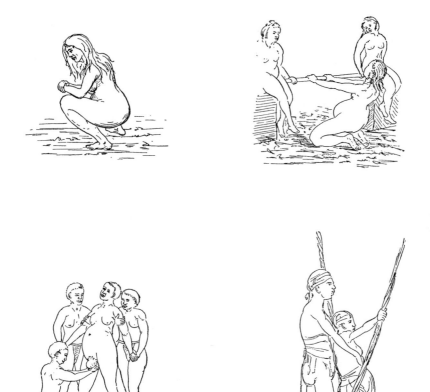

Source: George J. Engelman, *Labor among Primitive Peoples.* St. Louis: J. H. Chamber & Co., 1882.

have an easier and quicker passage through the pelvis and birth canal, movement is necessary. Lying in bed is detrimental to this process. Freedom of movement allows the laboring mother to instinctively get into any positions that facilitate the descent of the baby's head. I have watched women sway their hips rhythmically while in labor as if doing a slow belly dance. Women will go to their hands and knees, kneel, squat, sit, walk, stand, lean on a friend, or any other inventive movement that they can think of. The position that brings on stronger contractions may not always feel the best, nor does it comfort the pain of contractions. This is good; this is working hard to get the baby out in the best possible way.

Water helps make movement easier. Laboring on the land or on the bed is more difficult for the mother, for movement takes more effort. The buoyancy of the water supports the mother, requiring less effort on the mother's part to maintain a squatting position or a hands and knees position. The movement from one position to another can be a real chore out of the water. I felt like a beached whale while out of the tank when my midwives asked me to roll on my back in order to have a vaginal exam. Just the movement of changing positions in the water is easier than it is on land and far less energy consuming. The midwife needs to watch that the laboring mother's energy does not get drained from staying in the tank for too long. Some signs of the water draining the laboring mother of her energies are contractions slowing down and not lasting as long. The mother may feel that she wants to go to sleep or cannot keep her head up, even though she is not in real hard labor yet. Her cheeks may become flushed, and she may be perspiring a lot. This could be an indication that the water may be too hot for her or that she has been in the tank too long.

A woman will often get stuck in a position that feels good, where she can "stand" the pain, and may want to stay in that position for a long period of time. This, too, can delay the descent of the baby's head. Staying in one position for long periods of time (thirty to forty-five minutes) concerns me, for sometimes a cervical lip can form, preventing the mother from pushing when it is time to push.

Gravity assists in the decension of the baby's head due to the simple gravitational law that mass attracts mass. Squatting, especially while having a contraction, works superbly with the gravitational pull of the earth, one mass, attracting the other mass, the baby. It makes perfect sense either to stand or to squat in order to assist the baby's head in descending through the mother's pelvis and down through the birth canal. Working with gravity, abetted by a squatting position, opens the dimensions of the pelvis wider, with minimal muscle effort on the mother's part. The quantity of oxygen that is consumed is therefore less for both mother and baby. Squatting and using gravity is what our foremothers were taught to do by watching their mothers and sisters give birth. It has been part of our womanly tradition and is part of our heritage that we are reclaiming.

I am always impressed when I watch women shut down their intellect and use their intuition, especially first-time mothers. I remember Amanda, one of the first women whom I attended as a senior midwife. When the contractions got strong, Amanda needed no coaching. She simply got down on her haunches, in toad or frog position, and started bouncing around, as if from lily pad to lily pad. At first I thought this extremely strange; I had never seen anyone labor like this before. When I finally stopped making preconceived judgments, I realized the value of what Amanda was doing by putting double the amount of pressure into the pelvis through squatting and bouncing. Her labor was short and fairly easy. Amanda laughed afterward, saying that it was the best way she could figure out for getting the baby out. She said it felt good to feel the baby lower herself into the birth canal, which confirmed for Amanda that she was doing the right thing. This is what is called *active birth,* where the midwife supports the mother in making her own decisions as to when, how, and what is appropriate to help her labor progress.

As the labor progresses to 5 centimeters, the contractions become stronger, come closer (approximately three to five minutes apart), last longer (approximately thirty to forty-five seconds), and become increasingly intense. Remember the importance of relaxation, breathing, and surrender. The laboring mother will need someone to assist her with her breathing, reminding her to take the deep abdominal breaths and letting them out slowly through her open mouth and relaxed jaw. Staying in the birthing tank can help the mother relax. She should use whatever tools work to enable her to relax and let her body do what it needs to.

Remember to get in and out of the tank. Your body will know when to get out, just as you know when to get out of a hot bath or a hot tub. If your energy starts feeling drained, it may be time to get out and have a change of scenery. Go out for a walk with your partner. When a contraction comes, squat to get the baby down lower. This is very beneficial if your labor has been dragging on for hours. I don't care if you are in downtown Milwaukee, when that contraction comes on, squat! Eating lightly and drinking juices, teas, or water hourly is important to keep oneself hydrated.

Another way to promote a good labor is to have the lights low. Candles or lanterns provide a warm, glowing feeling that electric lights cannot begin to convey. Make sure, however, that the midwife can see well enough to do her work well. Having some candles by the tank as well as having a flashlight handy can provide good lighting. I have been at births as a photographer where the midwife softly sang songs to the laboring mother that sounded like lullabies, but when I listened closely to the words, the words were of strength and courage. One song that the mother can sing, which gives good visualizations, is: "I am a hollow bamboo tube, open for my babe to come through."

Many women will select music during their pregnancy that is soothing and relaxing to play during their labors. I had tapes of Debussy and Chopin made by my neighbor Steve Bradley just for the occasion. The music helped me with imagery, taking me to mythical places, with green grasses and huge old shade trees where lily of the valley grew all around. I could almost smell their beautiful fragrance. As labor became more intense, whale sounds were played for me. These sounds hit me in a very primal point. I felt very strong while listening to the whale sounds, as if I too were one of the ancient creatures. I imagined myself to be a whale, and the imagery connected me with my mammalian water cousins. It helped me to become more primal in my thinking, which encouraged me to let go more and allow my body to work as it should.

After the midway point, 5 centimeters, it may be harder to stay focused on relaxing. The midwife or the partner can help the mother remain oriented by keeping eye-to-eye contact with her and joining her in deep abdominal breathing. This deep abdominal breathing means breathing with the entire lungs, right down to the bottom of the rib cage. The lungs reach from the top of the rib cage to the very bottom. Inhale as deeply as you can and feel your lungs expand first from the bottom, through the middle of your chest, to the top of the lungs, and then slowly release. Some refer to this style of breathing as the Bradley method.

At this point, many women just want to stay in the tank. The relaxing properties of the warm water are supporting the laboring mother to the fullest extent. Use the water's buoyant properties to get into the different positions that will help get the baby out: squatting and holding on to the side of the tank or being supported by a friend or your partner. The hands and knees position helps to relieve the pressure off the back for a period of time, as does sitting on the bottom of the tank, leaning up against the inflatable water toys. A friend can splash water onto the exposed parts, such as the abdomen. I have found that even the splashing of the water on the belly can stimulate contractions. If you are one of those lucky enough to have a tank with jacuzzi jets, by all means use the jets on the parts of the body that are feeling discomfort. The jets can massage the lower back and other parts of the body very nicely. The belly can also be massaged by the jets, if they are not too forceful, which can be uncomfortable or may bring on stronger contractions. The water on the body reminds me of a water effleurage. Effleurage is the feathery touch of the hands on the mother's belly, which many women say feels wonderful—like the wings of an angel brushing against her belly. Effleurage also stimulates contractions.

At 5 to 8 centimeters the mother may want to stay in the tank for twenty to thirty minutes, lengthening the time in the water as the contractions become more intense. Then she may want to get out of the tank and move around. She may want to eat lightly if she can keep things down. Most women want to get back into the tank immediately, because the water reduces the pain. If labor at this point is moving along slowly, I ask the laboring mothers to move around. Remember to urinate while out of the tank. It is the job of the labor coach or the father to remind the mother to urinate every hour, so that the bladder is not full with the baby's head pushing against it. Sitting on the toilet also helps to get the baby further down into the birth canal. So stay there for a few minutes and relax. Remember to drink plenty of water while in labor, for the body is using up a lot of fluids and they need to be replenished. If you accidentally urinate in the tank, do not be alarmed since urine is sterile. Just do not make a habit of it, and try to make it to the toilet or chamber pot the next time.

At about 7 to 8 centimeters, the contractions will get closer (one to three minutes apart) and last as long as a minute. The baby is getting lower and lower in the birth canal. If your birth attendant isn't with you at this point, she should be. If she is not there, find your *Emergency Childbirth* book by Dr. Gregory White and have it close at hand. The midwife still has time to get there, but it is good to have the handbook close by in case things speed up. Being in the water now is almost a necessity. The laboring mother is heading toward transition and will not want to get out of the tank—the water just feels so good. At this point I encourage the mother to stay in the tank if this is what she desires.

Eventually, the contractions will come back to back, one on top of the other. At this point the mother is usually dilated 9 to 10 centimeters. This is called transition. This time between the laboring stage and the pushing stage can be very intense. Some mothers feel that they cannot go on anymore, they may want to go to the hospital, or they may ask for drugs. Transition can feel like such a helpless state, but it lasts only a short while—from a few minutes to a half hour. The water will help ease this time. I have seen some women, owing to the relaxing properties of the water, not even realize that they were in transition. When I told them that they were ready to push, they could not believe it, having prepared themselves for a longer and harder period.

During my own labor, I can remember what was going on in my head when I was in transition. I kept thinking that I really couldn't do this any longer. If I was only this far along, my God, what was the rest of labor going to be like? What had I been making all the laboring women do for all of these years? I felt that there was something wrong with me; I felt so inadequate. I couldn't lie on the bed or sit in the tank and calmly breathe like all the hundreds of women that I had seen give birth. Why couldn't I do this? My midwife gently reminded me that all women feel this way and that women have been giving birth since the beginning of time and have made it through. She reminded me that I was doing just what I needed to do—I was doing just fine—and that soon I would be able to push. I hung on to these words. My transition was very quick but *very* intense. I didn't labor the way I thought I was supposed to, but looking back, I labored the only way I knew how, the only way I could, which is the correct way.

At the point of transition, the most important thing to do is to empower oneself by surrendering to the forces of the labor. Know that transition only lasts a short time. Women do not die in childbirth as a result of the intensity of the labor; rarely do they die in childbirth at all. With calm, reassuring support, it is possible to get through this stage and start pushing when the cervix has completely effaced and dilated. The midwife or coach can be invaluable at this point in helping the laboring mother through a tough time. The laboring mother may feel that she cannot make it through this point or may feel that she can't go on. This feeling is a transition in itself. It is the ultimate surrender of oneself at this point—transition—the passage of pregnancy to active motherhood. Now mother and baby must do the final work to live as two individual human beings.

Elizabeth recalls how her midwife helped her through this final phase before pushing:

> I sat in the water with my back against the wall. My midwife sat beside me on the outside of the pool, coaching me through this last phase. I recall that she became my lifeline at this point. I trusted her to bring me and the baby through the force of the contractions without problems. The contractions were involutary, and it was this automatic sensation which I remember clearly. The force of each final contraction flowed through my body like a wave, each surge threatening to tear me apart. I watched the waves, unable to control them. It was due to my midwife that I allowed them to pass without increasing the force with conscious pushing. My midwife explained beforehand that I would have to watch her closely and follow her directions as the baby crowned in order to prevent tearing. It is essential that there is this trust, especially since the pain and intensity could cause fear.

At 9 to 10 centimeters, the mother often feels the urge to push. Grunting sounds and urges to move the bowels alert me to check the mother. I give her a vaginal exam at this point to see if she is completely dilated. The laboring mother must be complete, 10 centimeters, in order to push the baby out. The exam *can* be given in the water. If the midwife is in the tank with the mother, she can simply slide her hand into the vagina. If the midwife is not in the tank, then it is a bit more difficult, but the attendant can lean over the edge of the tank and give the exam that way. *There is no need to get the mother out of the tank.* At 10 centimeters, the cervix is said to be completely dilated and ready to push the baby out. There is such a well-earned sigh of relief at this point. All the hardest work is done, with just a little more work to do. Pushing.

K. Hansen, G. J. Hofmeyr, and L. Silcock of the Johannesburg Hospital and the University of the Witwatersrand in South Africa report that in a study of twelve women who gave birth in the water, they found that immersion in water was effective in helping women to relax during labor. They encouraged the mothers to enter the water bath when they felt ready to do so. Hansen et al. found that the water allowed each mother to be very mobile and to find the positions most comfortable for her. Sometimes it produced a state of extreme relaxation in which the mother seemed to be oblivious to her surroundings and less inhibited. They state that the purpose of their unit is not to promise uncomplicated childbirth, but to allow women to use their personal resources to achieve a fulfilling and positive birth experience.

One major role of a birth attendant is to encourage the mother to use her instincts as much as possible during labor. Many women, if encouraged, will begin to tap into a lower brain consciousness, a primal state where the thinking mind is not as dominant and women can then tune into their physical and emotional needs. It is a state of mind where the woman stops trying to control her body and surrenders to the innate sense of how to give birth. Often I see women trying to fight labor, trying to control it. When a woman releases her strong will, or stops fighting labor, she can get into an altered state of mind: a meditative state where she goes into the ancient *cellular* memory of knowing how to labor without having to think about it.

Linda K. Church, a nurse-midwife who attends water births at the Family Birthing Center in Upland, California, notes how women can relax without using medication and appear to experience less pain. She observes that there is a decrease in anxiety among women laboring in water. She hypothesizes that this is due to the reduction of adrenalin levels, which therefore encourages the release of the mother's natural oxytocins and endorphins.

Endorphins are produced while women are laboring, helping them cope with the pain of labor. These substances are like the woman's own opiates that the body produces. If the woman is tense or frightened, another chemical manufactured by the body will kick in. This is called adrenaline, which suppresses the endorphins. Oxytocin, a hormone produced by the mother's body that stimulates uterine contractions, is also suppressed by the adrenaline. The use of warm water assists in relaxation, alleviating fear and thus the production of adrenalin, allowing the oxytocin and endorphins to work to their fullest degree.

In "Catecholamines: The Effect of Maternal Fear and its Treatment on Uterine Function and Circulation," Gershon Levinson and Sol M. Shnider point out that "anxious mothers had weaker contractions and longer labors and higher circulating catecholamine levels" (1979, p. 167). Catecholamines cause the "fight or flight" responses, increased heart rate, increased blood pressure, constriction of the blood vessels, and other involuntary body responses.

"In animal studies," they write, "catecholamines resulted in lower uterine blood flow" and reduced heartbeat in the baby. They add that, when the uterine blood flow is reduced, the normal fetus has to work harder to get the oxygen needed, while a baby in trouble to begin with may not be able to get the oxygen it needs and could be liable to oxygen deprivation injury.

"In conclusion," write the doctors, "the evidence is that anxiety can increase maternal catecholamines. Catecholamines have the potential to deleteriously affect the mother and the fetus, and there are medications and techniques which will relieve that stress. We believe that, given a very anxious and stressed mother, we are not helping the baby by not relieving the stress. Preferably, the stress should be relieved nonpharmacologically" (p. 173).

Levinson and Shnider show the importance of the mother being relaxed and comfortable with her body, both for the effectiveness of labor and for the health of the baby during labor. Some women may find it difficult to attune to this birth instinct. Some silent time by herself, with the lights lowered and a favorite piece of music playing, can give the mother the chance to relax and surrender to the course of labor within her. The mother's feelings and desires take precedence during labor, which is another good reason why laboring women need to take some time for introspection. This is well accomplished in the tank of water. I generally let the mother decide when to enter the tank. If she asks when to get in, I tell her whenever she feels like it. The laboring mother will know what to do. I find that most women cannot wait to get in and may be waiting only because they aren't sure when is the correct time. By asking the mother what appeals to her, the birth attendant reaffirms the primacy of the mother's instincts and her innate ability to know the appropriate time to enter the tank. My rule is: the appropriate time to enter the water is the time that feels right to the mother. Women know what to do while in labor. We need to reclaim our sense of self-authority, of self-governance, especially when it comes to pregnancy and birth.

RELAXATION IN LABOR

Nature's hands are never so obviously active as during labor, and a woman in labor alone knows their strength. When she is relaxed, the muscles in her body are free to follow their ancient patterns as life begets life. Relaxation can be accomplished in a variety of ways. I en-

courage the woman during her pregnancy to find what method of relaxation works for her, to become familiar with it, and to include it as
part of her daily life.

During my pregnancy I got a massage as often as possible. I found
this worked well to relax the muscles that were carrying all the extra
weight. I often massage women or encourage their partners to massage
them while they are in labor. The response to the massage is almost
immediate relaxation. Certain parts of the body tense up while in labor.
Be aware of where the tension is held. Areas that tend to get tight are
the buttocks and thighs and the neck and shoulders. When an area
appears to be tense, reminding the mother to "relax your face" or "relax
your hands" can help with this surrender. If she has problems locating
the areas, touching the woman's body can help her locate the spots
where the tenseness needs to be released.

I found with my own labor that the use of hydrojets was extremely
helpful in assisting me to relax. At St. Luke's Medical Center in Denver,
Colorado, Kathleen Aderhold and Leslie Perry have assisted women
who used jet hydrotherapy while in labor. They were impressed how
tense muscles were able to relax due to the massaging of the hydrojets.
Even the nipples of the mothers were able to be massaged, stimulating
the release of oxytocin and thus bringing on stronger contractions. They
also found that the jets relieved back labor and could give a good massage to many tense areas of the body.

There are different schools of thought on how to breathe while in
labor. The breathing that I have observed to support the mother best
for relaxation is the Bradley method, which is essentially a deep abdominal breathing. Relaxation lends itself to a less painful, easier,
quicker birth. The mind needs to relax and let the body do the work.
In my practice, I have not seen the Lamaze method work nearly as
well. I have not seen it being conducive to relaxation, but for shifting
one's concentration to somewhere else. The breathing method seems to
work in the very early stages of labor, but when hard labor hits, the
laboring mother does not need to be concentrating on getting the right
breathing pattern down. I can remember arriving at the home of several couples who were attempting the Lamaze method, who were in a
frenzy because they couldn't remember if they were supposed to blow
or puff or pant at that point. One laboring mother was so uptight that
her eyes were bulging and her fists were clenched. I sat her down in a
rocker and encouraged her to rock in a slow and easy pattern. Then we
started breathing together, taking deep abdominal breaths through the
nose, and exhaling through the mouth, letting the jaw hang loose.
Every muscle in her body started to relax, and she began to smile. Some
believe that the jaw is connected to the cervix, and if the jaw is relaxed,
the cervix will be too, enabling quicker dilation. It stands to reason that

if all other parts of the body are relaxed, the cervix will be also and therefore able to open better.

Another way to relax while in labor is through meditation. There are numerous ways to meditate. Simply clear your mind of any thoughts. Do the meditation that was described in Chapter 4 or one you have been using during your pregnancy. Get in touch with your baby. Send him or her your love and strength. Try to convey that the two of you can do this together. In your stillness, feel the spirit of the child. Find your inner strength. Become centered and let your body take over and do what it needs to do.

While assisting laboring women, many times I have seen them get overwhelmed by the thought of the contractions becoming more intense. Reminding them to stay focused on that particular contraction always seems to help them remain calm. Helping them stay in the moment, and not to think about what the next contractions are going to be like, is of great assistance. I have used the analogy of a contraction to a wave to help women get through contraction after contraction. The connection with water also seems to be soothing, especially for someone who is having a water birth. The imagery goes like this: "In your mind's eye, see the contraction building, like a wave. Let the wave take you. Ride the wave. As its strength crests, let it take you and caress you while you sit high on that wave. Then the wave slowly and gently meets the shore, putting you softly on the beach to wait for the next wave to catch and ride again with strength." I find that visualizations are also an important key to surrendering to the forces of one's body. I tell women to visualize themselves as a hollow bamboo tube that opens up for the baby to come through. I encourage them to see the baby coming down the tube and to imagine one's self getting looser and opening wider. Images of a head coming through a turtleneck sweater or the petals of a flower unfolding one by one, revealing the baby's head, can help in the dilation of the cervix.

The mind is very powerful, and many women have found the value of doing visualizations while in labor. I remember one woman who used this tool very well. Her bag of waters broke at dawn. I was staying in a little cabin close to her house, so it was just a minute's walk for her husband to come and get me. His big radiant smile told me something was going on, and I didn't have to guess what. The morning smells were fresh, the sun was weaving her golden threads through the sky. It was a beautiful day to have a baby. Paula, the laboring mother, looked as radiant as the morning. She lay on the bed next to the tank, breathing deeply. "How ya doing?" I asked. "Just great!" she beamed back. As a contraction came on, she continued breathing and appeared to go into a deep meditative state. When the contraction was over, she looked at me and remarked how well the imagery and visualizations were working for her. In the background soft lulling music was playing, music that she had listened to during her pregnancy, music that was familiar to her.

Another contraction. I guided her through this one with the image of a rosebud opening petal by petal. There is your baby's face in the middle of the flower, I said. That is your baby's head coming through the cervix. Paula had worked with guided imagery and visualizations throughout her pregnancy. She also used positive affirmations in her daily life. One of her affirmations was, "I am totally surrendering to my body's forces, knowing that it will do what it needs to do." After assessing the whole situation and assuring myself that Paula was doing well, I decided to give them time alone. Her husband, John, helped her with deep breathing as he massaged her. Expecting an entire day's labor, since Paula was a first-time Mom and her bag of waters had just broken two hours before, I sat in the next room. When I checked in, Paula was lying on the bed making grunting noises like those of a woman pushing. "Hey, it's too early for that," I said, while looking between her legs at her vulva. I could see a quarter's worth of the baby's head! "Get into the tank or you're going to have this baby on your bed," I said. John came rushing into the tank with us. Two hours later, after some pushing, Camilla was born.

Although Paula's first stage of labor did not take place in the tank, she had an amazingly fast first stage. I attribute this to her ability to use the tools of visualization, imagery, and affirmations to help empower herself to relax.

I have received a videotape from my Russian friends. In this video, a midwife, Tanya, is shown giving birth to her third child. I was struck by the confidence this woman had in herself and her body. She was in charge but did not try to control. I watched as she squatted in the tank alone, her husband reading poetry to her. Gregorian chants played in the background. She was surrendering to the forces of her labor. Never had I seen a mother so relaxed, and at the same time, Tanya was doing her own perineal massage. The baby's head popped out, she gave a little grunt, and pushed out the rest of the baby into the water. Tanya smiled serenely as she lifted her daughter from the water, welcoming her with kisses into the new world. I thought to myself that every woman has the capability to give birth with such power and grace.

When I'm attending a woman in labor, I remind her of the miracle that is going on in her body, the miracle of another human being coming from her body. This doesn't happen every day—perhaps once in a lifetime. Step outside of your body, I tell her, put your mind on the ceiling, and watch what your body can do. The bodily function of birth is at the least physiologically interesting and at the most miraculous. Tell your body, "Take me and do what you need to do. I trust in you." Through empowerment comes the ability to surrender. To surrender to child-birth, the woman must be confident that her body knows what to do and trust it.

To remember and use these keys to relaxation is quite an accomplish-ment when a woman is in the throes of a hard contraction. But if the mother can be guided by her labor coach to think of the contraction as a wave, building slowly, reaching a crest, and fading to a gentle end, the contraction will be more friendly. I like this image of a wave. I tell her to ride it and let it take her. Give no resistance. Let the wave carry you and set you gently on the beach.

The contractions are a means to an end—to the birth of that baby. Relaxation, along with water, is one of the chief ways to make the con-tractions work as effectively as possible. No synthetic pain killers are necessary, nor are synthetic oxytocins necessary to bring on labor. With the help of water combined with one's own mind and intuition, the laboring mother's body will work efficiently.

In 1986, while doing research on underwater births, I visited with Dr. Serge Wesel at the Hospital de Braine l'Alleud–Waterloo in Bel-gium, where laboring in the water was made available at the woman's request. Although Dr. Wesel did not permit women to give birth in the tanks, first-stage labor in warm water was found to be very effective. Dr. Wesel has been assisting women to labor in water since 1982. I found the tank to be the size of a large European bathtub. Close by was a bed to give birth on when the time was ripe. Oxygen tanks were right beside the bed concealed by pillows. Other emergency equipment was also available in the room in case the need arose. All in all, the room had the appearance of a hospital room, except for the labor tank. The atmosphere in the hospital was inviting, with original drawings and weavings of pregnant women, birth, and women with children. Dr. We-sel spoke encouragingly of his experience of water labor; "The bath had a relaxing, a reassuring and analgesic effect which provided favorable conditions for a satisfactory delivery. The bath's effect could enable women to master the pain and also to relax and find comfort in reas-suring figures such as their partners and their mothers, and to regress sufficiently to be responsive to their babies" (Boulvain and Wesel, 1985).

Dr. Wesel conducted a study of eighteen women. All had to be in active labor, have regular contractions, ruptured membranes, and di-lated to at least 4 centimeters. The study showed that mothers were more available to welcome the child; the bath might facilitate primary maternal preoccupation, as well as a greater desire to communicate and to create contact with the baby. The *sage-femmes* (midwives) in the hospital were also supportive of water labor and were anxious to exchange information. At the time, it was one of the few hospitals in the world that was advocating the use of warm water while in labor. I found it encouraging that medical establishments were starting to recognize the value of water for laboring.

EATING AND DRINKING WHILE IN LABOR

Another way to make contractions work efficiently is to eat properly while in labor. Our bodies need fuel to work effectively, and this is even more true in labor. The body is working very hard. I give my mothers protein smoothies made of bananas, fresh fruit, protein powder, egg yolk, water, brewers yeast, and wheat germ. Anything may be added or subtracted according to the mother's palate. Miso soup with vegetables is wonderfully nourishing. I like to keep a pot simmering on the stove. It can be enjoyed by everyone during the labor and after the birth as well. Eat food that is easy to digest. Stay away from meat and dairy products. Eat whole foods, such as fresh fruit, vegetables, or grains, and have nothing refined. It is best to eat while in early labor. Once the body gets into harder labor, digestion slows down. Not many mothers care to eat in the later stages of labor.

Laboring mothers need to drink plenty of water, juices, and teas. Certain fruit juices replenish the body's electrolytes, such as Knudsen's Recharge. It is extremely important to be well hydrated during labor, for the body is constantly manufacturing amniotic fluid and perspiring from the hard work and from immersion in a tank of warm water. Lost electrolytes need to be replaced if muscles are to work properly. Kathleen Aderhold and Leslie Perry studied water births and found that sitting in warm baths during labor increased diuresis (increased secretion of urine). Other studies conducted by doctors and midwives have made similar observations. Please keep a lot of fluids running through the laboring mother, and don't forget to urinate at least once an hour.

OTHER CONSIDERATIONS

As anyone who has been in a hot tub knows, one can't stay in over an extended period of time; one gets in and out. Laboring too long in water can drain one's energy. Besides, it is good to get out and walk around, and perhaps go outdoors. Sometimes just changing the scenery can change the whole energy of the labor and further it along.

Walking enables the body to work with the pull of gravity in order to lower the baby into the pelvis. Going for a good long walk and squatting during the contractions helps the baby's head engage and the labor to progress. Moving the body is necessary in labor for this very reason. If, after walking, the head is still high and needs to engage, several things can be done. I have found that getting into the water and squatting during a contraction is effective. The water is relaxing for the mother, and squatting takes less effort in the water.

If there are still problems with the progression of the labor, I have heard of women taking a half cup to a cup of herbal teas such as Blue Cohosh (*Caulophyllum thalictroides*), Black Cohosh (*Cimicifuga race-mosa*), or Pennyroyal (*Hedeoma pulegioides*). Any or all of these com-bined can help to stimulate the pituitary gland, which in turn releases the oxytocin that stimulates labor. Not more than half a cup should be taken as titanic contractions can occur, which could compromise the health of the baby. All of these herbs are good to have at hand before labor starts. Consult with your doctor or midwife before taking any of these herbs. *Note: These herbs are not to be taken during the pregnancy as they can induce a miscarriage.*

INFORMATION FOR THE BIRTH ATTENDANT

The birth attendant's equipment needs to be as close to the tank as possible. I usually ask the couple to provide a small table next to the tank which is easily accessible. Emergency equipment needs to be close at hand and can be placed on the table. One of my instruments is a doppler, which works on ultrasound and monitors the baby's heartbeat. Using any form of ultrasound is still controversial. The method has not been around long enough to be proven safe. However, I do carry an ultrasound doppler for questionable times when it's difficult to find the fetal heart tones. It is almost impossible to use a fetoscope—a type of stethoscope used to listen to the baby's heartbeat—under water. To use a fetoscope, the mother's hips may be raised out of the water. At times, the fetal heart tones cannot be immediately found. It can be uncom-fortable for the mother to be raised out of the water in this awkward position over any length of time. I have found that a Parks doppler, if used sparingly, can be a great asset in water births. It has a remote lead that can be immersed in the water without having to raise the woman's hips. The unit can be flashed on for fifteen seconds, just long enough to get an idea of how the fetal heart tones are doing in between, during, or after a contraction.

I like to listen to the baby's heartbeat once every hour or more often as indicated, until transition. I then monitor more frequently, such as every ten minutes. Once the mother starts pushing, I monitor after every contraction. Normally, the baby's heartbeat ranges from 120 to 160 beats per minute (BPM). If the BPM starts swinging too much, such as 100 to 180, then I will ask the mother to get out of the water to assess what the problem is.

Previously, I used a Medsonics doppler, which is one solid unit (elec-tronics and transmitter). This unit cannot be immersed in water, however. The woman's hips need to be raised out of the water, but only for fifteen seconds or so to get an accurate fetal heart tone reading. This particular doppler was once immersed in water, and problems arose with the doppler. Birth attendants should therefore be careful to keep this kind of equipment dry when attending water births. One doctor proposed putting a surgical glove or condom over it, but I have never tried it.

Taking the blood pressure can be done in the tank or out. I have noticed that if the laboring mother's blood pressure is up, the water helps to lower it. After studying thirty-one low-risk women, Myra Smith found that the mean aterial pressure and anxiety level signifi-cantly decreased after fifteen minutes in the tub and remained reduced (1987). In another study, Christine Brown found that during the first few minutes after immersion, the blood pressure would increase slightly, but then after a few minutes it would decrease and stay de-creased (1982).

A clean bed or mat with a plastic liner under a sterile sheet should be right next to the tank. Then the mother may easily move from bed to tank and vice versa. Should there be an emergency, or should labor in the water need to be stopped, the mother can easily be transported to the bed.

Getting in and out of the tank brings foreign matter into the water. This matter is anything that can be dragged in on the feet or the rest of the body. Even lint carries bacteria. Although the chance of infection is lower in the home than in the hospital or birthing clinic, extra meas-ures of cleanliness are worthwhile. I advise anyone who is entering the tank to wash off with a betadine solution or tincture of green soap, paying close attention to the feet and hands. It is wise to have a dish pan on the outside of the tank that contains a 50 percent betadine and 50 percent water solution so that everyone entering the tank can rinse their feet. The tank itself should be scrubbed with the full-strength solution each time before filling it with water.

One of the main complaints that I have heard from women who have had a hospital birth is the routine administration of an enema. I feel that giving an enema, unless requested by the mother, is an intrusion. Besides, most women find that their bodies naturally start evacuating themselves a few days before labor begins, leaving only small amounts of feces in the colon. When I first started attending water births, one of the main concerns was infection due to feces being passed during the pushing stage. To remedy this possibility, I give women enemas when they reach about 5 centimeters dilation. I wait until 5 centimeters be-cause I encourage women to eat in the early stages of labor. Usually at the halfway point of the first stage, most women do not want to eat, so that is a good time to administer the enema, cleaning the colon before the pushing stage. If a bit of feces are passed during pushing, the pooper scooper (aquarium fish net) is able to catch most of the droppings that get into the tank. An important point to remember is that often after getting an enema and vacating the bowels, stronger labor can strongly and rapidly kick in. I ask my pregnant mothers to wait until the midwife is there before taking an enema.

PREMATURE RUPTURE OF THE AMNIOTIC SAC

There is one exception to the rule of intuiting the time of immersing oneself in the tank: if labor begins with the rupture of her bag of waters and if after an hour or so there is no sign of labor (that is, contractions have not begun), it may be best to stay out of the tank. Signs of true labor usually start showing within the first three hours after the water breaks. It is true labor when the contractions get progressively stronger, last longer, and come closer together. They do not stop. As a general rule, labor should be steadily progressing for several hours after the bag of waters has broken—the assurance that true labor is underway—before the mother enters the tank. If true labor has already been determined by rhythmic contractions, the laboring mother may get into the tank when she instinctively feels like it.

At a birth center named Sodersjukhuset in Stockholm, Sweden, Ulla Waldenstrom and Carl-Axel Nilsson compared eighty-nine women who labored in water after spontaneous rupture of the membranes to eighty-nine women who did not labor in water after the waters broke. They found no statistical difference between the groups regarding infections, respiratory problems in the newborn, or asphyxia, nor were there any signs of maternal amnionitis. The study also showed that the Apgar scores of the newborn were lower at five minutes in the group that bathed. The researchers found that there was an association between the length of time the bag of waters (ruptured membranes) were broken and the low Apgar score (longer than twenty-four hours). They also questioned the interval of time as to when the first vaginal exam was given. As a rule, when the membranes break, I will not do vaginal exams until good hard labor has been present for a few hours or until I need to determine if it is time to push. With the Apgar scoring, a slight deviation from the standard scoring system needs to take place, for the Apgar scoring was designed for babies born in hospitals with routine hospital occurrences.

The only time I ask the laboring mother not to enter the tank is when the membranes rupture prematurely. If the water breaks prematurely, the woman may not be physiologically ready to go into labor, but she is now technically in labor. This early rupture may be due to too great physical exertions. The bag of waters can also break when the sac is pinched between the baby's head and the pelvic bones. There are numerous other reasons for an early rupture as well.

A main concern of practitioners for women laboring and birthing in the water is infection. Kathleen Aderhold and Leslie Perry (1991) attended women with ruptured membranes who labored in water without any signs of infection. They felt that ruptured membranes alone were not a good reason to restrict tub use, and they found that there was no increase of infection. They also cultured the tanks, finding that as long as the tanks were well cleaned (they used chlorine bleach and turned on the jets for water circulation), there was no increase in organism count.

Once the water breaks, the mother and the baby are open to infection, because bacteria can now get into the uterus. Occasionally, women will not go into labor for days after an early rupture. Vaginal exams are then out of the question, for anything put into the vagina can introduce bacteria, even when a sterile glove is used. The practitioner and couple need to watch for signs of uterine infection if after twenty-four hours the pregnant mother has not gone into labor. These signs include (1) the mother's body temperature rising to 100° F and above; (2) pulse becoming weaker with a rate increase of at least 20 beats per minute higher than her normal rate; (3) any foul smells that may be coming from the vagina; (4) meconium; and (5) blood test for elevated white blood cell count.

Thomas B. Lebherz et al. (1960) reported that in a "typical" hospital labor, while infection after premature rupture could occur, it was not very common. In a study of 787 women with premature ruptures, the infection rate in the first three days was about 7 out of 1,000. From four days on, the rate jumped to about 40 infections per 1,000 premature ruptures.

Most practitioners want to see signs of hard labor within twenty-four to seventy-two hours. After this amount of time, the chances of infection increase. If true labor has not begun by twenty-four hours after the water breaks, I like to reassess the situation and consult with my backup doctor to determine if the laboring mother needs to go to the hospital.

After the membranes rupture, I like to see the contractions developing a true labor pattern before I encourage a woman to get into the water. Most women tend to start contractions almost immediately after the water breaks or the waters break due to the contractions.

Sometimes contractions do not start up for hours. I have found this to be a phenomenon more common among first-time mothers. If she feels very strongly about getting into the tank, I will respect her intuition, for water may be the trick to relaxation and getting her into labor. However, I advise her to relax in a warm shower instead of the tank because a shower poses no threat of infection. After the rupture, amniotic fluid usually trickles periodically from the vagina, but occasionally, the membranes will stop leaking. I then question if the amniotic sac actually did break or whether instead the vagina is excreting the mother's juices, getting her ready for labor. Periodically, the mother may have uncontrolled urination, owing to the baby's head moving down, putting pressure against the bladder. Urine can also be mistaken for rupture of the membrane. The practitioner or the pregnant mother can have nitrazine paper on hand, which can be obtained from the pharmacy. The paper can be placed in the fluid to determine whether or not the discharge is amniotic fluid. If it is amniotic fluid, the paper will turn a dark blue. (The pH of amniotic fluid is alkaline.)

The classic gush of water usually alerts the mother to the onset of labor. What if this happens, but then it stops leaking? On occasion, there is a tear high in the amniotic sac (maybe in the upper region of the mother's abdominal area), which allows enough amniotic fluid to escape for the baby's head to descend lower into the pelvis. The baby's head can act like a cork, stopping the flow of amniotic fluid. It is reassuring to know that amniotic fluid replenishes itself as long as the mother is keeping herself well hydrated. If amniotic leakage stops and contractions slow or stop, the onset of labor may be many hours or even days away, and I would advise staying out of the tank.

During my research and study of underwater births I came across a very thorough and intriguing article in the *Journal of Nurse-Midwifery* by Christine Brown (1982), in which she lays out the basis of the therapeutic effects of a warm water tub for a laboring mother.

First, Brown points out that water is unsurpassed for carrying heat to all parts of the immersed body and that the buoyancy of water relieves the weight that the pregnant mother carries during the last trimester. But then she observes another effect of immersion: that the weight of the water exerts a pressure on the surface of the body.

"In order to maintain its equilibrium," she writes, "the body responds by shifting blood from the interior body core to the body surface" (p. 14). Just under the surface of the skin are sweat glands and capillaries controlled by the sympathetic nervous system, which responds to psychological as well as physical changes.

The flight-or-fight response is one such psychological change and produces profound effects on sweat produced and blood flow. A much more benign and relaxing response occurs when the skin is immersed in warm water and blood flows to the skin—a "soothing action on the cutaneous nerve endings and all organs with which the skin is in reflex connection" (p. 14), she writes, that is, on the entire sympathetic nervous system.

Brown states that since the veins are thinner and more easily com-

pressed than the arteries, the pressure of heavy water on the soft muscles of the body surface at first presses on the veins, increasing the rate
at which they return blood to the heart, and increases the venous blood
pressure. But the thermal effect of the warm water soon causes these
vessels to dilate, and blood more easily flows through them.

That is why "a transient increase in blood pressure is often seen at
the beginning of a warm bath, followed by a slight decrease in blood
pressure, with a strengthening of cardiac action and lowering of the
pulse rate," she writes. "These effects all reflect normal adaptation of
the body. There is no undue strain on the cardiovascular or nervous
system" (p. 15).

Brown also notes an increase in the amount of urine excreted by the
kidneys and a reduction in its acidity. In addition, "buoyancy of the
water counteracts the weight of the body on pressure areas. The relief
and feeling of weightlessness enhance the psychological relaxation a
person is able to achieve and cause a generalized relief of mental tension" (p. 15), she states. This is a wonderful but simple and available
technique for assisting laboring mothers to relax and enjoy the experience of birth.

There are yet more benefits. Brown maintains that the fatigue of
labor is reduced when the mother is more relaxed, as when she labors
in a relaxing tub of warm water, because undue muscular activity is
reduced. "The uterus and surrounding layers of abdominal muscle are
acutely sensitive to pressure during labor. If a woman tenses her abdominal muscles during a contraction, the pain of the contraction will
increase" (p. 15). The buoyancy of the water assists the woman by diminishing the pressure of the abdominal muscles on the uterus, thus
diminishing pain. After the contraction ends, the water helps the
mother relax and gather more strength for the next contraction. When
the muscles of the body are relaxed, Brown says, "the uterus is able to
contract more efficiently, and oxygenation of the laboring uterus and
removal of waste and products of metabolism occur more readily" (p.
15).

As athletes know, hydrotherapy is effective for pain relief. This analgesic effect is due to the superior ability of water to conduct heat,
especially when the water is kept at about 100 degrees—the temperature of blood and the deep tissues of the body. According to many
studies, hydrotherapy is effective in treating unlocalized pain associated with intestinal disorders or with the sympathetic nervous system.
As Brown points out, "Pain in the first stage of labor stems largely from
the uterus where sensory innervation is derived primarily from the
sympathetic nervous system" (p. 14).

High body temperatures, such as from fevers or saunas, have been
implicated as a possible teratogen during the first trimester when the

baby's organs are being formed. While taking a sauna exposes the body to temperatures of 175° to 194° F, "a warm bath equalizes the core temperature and that of the skin and subcutaneous tissues, but does not elevate the core temperature. Even with exposure of the mother to excess heat during the latter half of pregnancy, no adverse fetal effects have been found, so warm tub bathing during labor can be safely used" (p. 14).

Looking back to the first water birth that I attended, I was happy to find some of the points that Brown discussed. The temperature of the amniotic fluid is approximately 100° F. Rennie labored in that water temperature and found it to be too hot, consequently, draining her of her energy. We poured in a few buckets of cold water and cooled the tank down to about 99° F. This seemed to work better for Rennie, and she was able to stay in the water longer without being zapped of her energy. Another discovery we made during this labor was that her husband, Larry, designed the tank too deep. When Rennie sat on the bottom of the tank, the water was just below her chin. She found this too deep, making her feel claustrophobic. We brought in a stool for her to sit on, and this brought the water level to right above her breasts. Sighing with relief, Rennie relaxed once more and continued with her labor. I found that this water level was also comfortable for women in the subsequent water births that I attended.

COMPLICATIONS DURING THE FIRST STAGE OF LABOR

Laboring in water has many benefits for the laboring mother, as I have already shown. I have found that water can also remedy complications that occur during labor. I have seen women whose blood pressure became too high due to the stress of labor. Soon after they get into the water they relax, and the blood pressure goes down to its normal range. I have also observed that a baby that is presenting in an occiput posterior (the head is facing up, looking at the mother's abdomen, instead of facing down) position can rotate spontaneously to the less difficult delivery of occiput anterior, the position that is most favorable for delivery, face down, if the mother has greater ability to move freely. The difficulty with the posterior presentation is that labor is usually longer, and laboring mothers may suffer with severe back labor since the baby's spine and back of the head are pressing against the mother's spine. The baby's spine is usually lined up against the mother's abdomen.

During my practice with water births, not all of them have been completed in the water. As with any labor or delivery, complications do arise that may necessitate going to the hospital or continuing with a traditional home delivery. I have found that in most instances if labor cannot continue in the water, then it is not appropriate to continue at home. Yes, there may be periods when the laboring mother needs to stay out of the water, but when the problems have been corrected, labor can continue in the water. If the problems cannot be corrected by staying out of the water, then the midwife needs to assess whether or not it is necessary to go to the hospital.

One of the most common reasons I have encountered for not continuing with a water birth is failure of the labor to progress. If after hours and hours of laboring, the woman is at the same centimeter of dilation as she was hours ago, it may be time for a reassessment. If laboring in the water doesn't help dilation, then she should get out of the water and squat or move around. Perhaps the mother may just need to rest. Carol experienced just that. She had labored most of the afternoon and on through the night. She had eaten during the early part of her labor and seemed to have plenty of energy throughout the day and most of the night. After midnight she began petering out. Her contractions slowed down and almost completely stopped, except for one every fifteen to twenty minutes. She was approximately 7 to 8 centimeters dilated and should have been having strong contractions every two minutes. She was tired and said that she did not like staying up so late. We gave her a smoothie with some honey in it for energy which just nauseated her. Carol lived by the Pacific Ocean, which that night was reflecting a beautiful full moon. After going for a walk and listening to the waves beating on the shore, my assistant told her that it was time to take a nap. We all went back into the house and helped Carol to lie down. We softly rubbed her head and did calming visualizations to get her to sleep. And sleep she did, for over an hour! She woke up with strong contractions. Three hours later she delivered a beautiful baby girl in the water.

If Carol had not been able to get back into hard labor, we would have gone to the hospital. Laboring moms who run out of energy can sometimes have problems with hemorrhaging. For example, it is sometimes harder for the uterus to expel the placenta after the delivery of the baby, as the uterus can become "boggy" and unable to contract to shut off the open vessels at the former placental site. The baby may also be getting worn out and stressed, which can compromise the safety of the baby, especially if the pushing stage is difficult. With this in mind, if a laboring mother is running out of energy and the labor has been going on for days, it may be best to complete the labor in the hospital.

Meconium

Fetal heart tones, or the baby's normal heartbeat range, is 120 to 160 beats per minute. When the beats start deviating from this range, I start questioning what the problem could be and how to remedy it. I then ask the mother to get out of the water for several reasons. The first one is to evaluate if there is any meconium staining. Meconium is the baby's feces that are released if the baby is under stress. Meconium can only be detected if the membranes have ruptured, and usually, with a contraction, the amniotic fluid will run out of the mother's vagina. The fluid will either be clear or tinged with a yellow or green color, which indicates meconium. If I see any coloration of the fluid, I will ask the mother to stay out of the water through at least a half hour's worth of contractions to determine whether or not meconium is being passed and to see if the fetal heartbeat returns to the normal range. If there is light yellow or light green meconium, I advise the mother to stay out of the water. I monitor the color of the meconium until it is time to make a decision as to whether or not to transport to the hospital.

Watching the color of meconium in the tank is impossible. I keep a close watch on the fetal heartbeat, monitoring the beat every five minutes. I pay especially close attention to the fetal heartbeat immediately after a contraction to see how the baby responds to a contraction. If the baby passes thick pea soup meconium, then I start preparing to go to the hospital. If the bag of waters is not broken and the heartbeat is still swinging out of the range, then the laboring mother should lie down on her left side in her bed, and I monitor the fetal heart tones every five minutes. Another reason to get the mother out of the tub is to determine whether the waters have broken while in the water. The mother can sometimes feel the break of the sac, or particles of the vernix (the white cold cream-like covering on the baby's skin) can be seen floating in the tank's water. Occasionally, the baby will be born in the caul (the amniotic sac), which is truly an incredible sight to see. It is like seeing a precious jewel sparkling in the water. This is absolutely fine and can be broken after half a minute.

One midwife told me of a birth that resulted in the mother getting a strep infection. Strep had been going through the family; the mother had gotten it, and so had her two daughters. Everyone was completely over it, except the father who refused to get a culture. On the day the mother went into labor, he had a sore throat. Before the midwife arrived, the father had been giving the mother vaginal exams without any gloves on. After the mother climbed into the tank to continue her labor, he also got into the tank. It isn't clear whether the strep was transmitted to the mother through the vaginal exams or because the father climbed into the tank with her. Anyone who is sick or has any cuts should not be in the tank. Nothing is worth taking risks that could be easily avoided.

Estimating Blood Loss

Estimating blood loss is hard to do while in the water. If enough blood is coming out of the laboring mother's vagina to discolor the water, get out of the tank immediately and watch for more blood coming with the next contraction. If the blood is light spotting or just a tablespoon's worth, it may be that the cervix is dilating and breaking vessels. If there is more than a tablespoon, the midwife should listen to the baby's heartbeat. If the fluctations are out of the normal range, a further evaluation by the midwife may be necessary, for there could be complications with the placenta. The woman should stay out of the tank, and the amount of blood loss should be monitored by the midwife for half an hour to an hour, depending on how much blood there is and how the heart tones are doing, to rule out the possibility of early placental separation or a low-lying placenta.

Cervical Lips

Occasionally, a cervical lip will form while laboring. A cervical lip is an edematous cervix. I sometimes explain it as a puffy cervix—a cervix where the blood flow has been cut off and remains trapped in the cervix unable to move. This usually happens toward the end of labor when the baby's head descends low into the birth canal and pinches the cervix between itself and the symphysis pubis. This situation often occurs when the mother finds a comfortable position while laboring, a position where she says "this position feels good, it doesn't hurt," and consequently she doesn't move for a long time.

A cervical lip is not unusual during labor, but it can be prevented if the woman changes her positions frequently. Before I attended water births, I would massage the cervix to get the circulation moving. This, as well as getting the mother in a hands-and-knees position, always seemed to help to get the baby's head off of the symphysis pubis. Unfortunately, the cervical lip usually occurs soon before the mother is ready to push, at about 9 centimeters. At this point in labor, getting into the hands and knees position is uncomfortable for many women. With a water birth the mother is able to stretch out on her back, thanks to the water buoyancy; she is able to float, putting less pressure on the venae cava. (The venae cava is the venous trunk receiving blood from the lower extremities and the pelvic region.) Many women complain that if they lie on their backs too long in the latter months of their pregnancy, they become uncomfortable. Also, lying on one's back is a big taboo whether it be at home or in the hospital. This is due to the weight of the baby pressing on the venae cava; when one is lying on one's back, the circulation of the blood to and from the uterus—and thus to the baby—is restricted.

When women lie on their backs, the baby's head moves away from the symphysis pubis. Massaging her cervix, preventing the blood from pooling, and getting it flowing can easily be achieved in the water and while the mothers are on their backs. The combination of the two is truly remarkable, and the cervix loses its edema faster than I had previously witnessed in other women.

Why can't the laboring mother simply wait out the cervix until the swelling goes down? The problem is that this usually happens toward the end of the first stage of labor when the mother has an intense urge to push. For some, the urge is absolutely uncontrollable. Since the cervix is swollen, filled with blood that cannot circulate well, the mother's pushing the baby onto the cervical lip can cause the mother to tear her cervix, causing heavy bleeding. She would then need to go to the hospital to have her cervix stitched up. It seems like a lot of hassle when all that is needed is a good coach to help the laboring mother to blow with short, quick breaths, which prevents her from pushing, along with good eye-to-eye contact, keeping the mother focused on the work that she needs to be doing, not closing her eyes and getting swallowed up by the intensity of the birth. When it is time to push, the cervix slips back over the baby's head as the baby decends lower into the birth canal. In a sense it disappears.

PRIORITIES

In the early years of my experience with water births, some parents confused priorities while in labor. It became apparent when complications surfaced and it was time to go to the hospital that a few people did not want to go because they were too attached to the idea of having a water birth. I have run across the same sort of people in traditional homebirths who were attached to having a homebirth beyond everything else. These people are "keeping up with the Joneses," so to speak, they usually have had friends who have had a successful water birth, and they want the same. Perhaps for some reason they feel that they will lose face and will be failures, or the idea is so locked into their belief systems that they cannot think straight. I must reiterate time and again that *the desired outcome for having a water birth is a healthy mother and baby*. These people are gambling with their lives and their babies' lives. I discuss with them the dangerous outcomes of staying at home when such complications arise. On one occasion when the couple insisted on staying at home, even after knowing that the baby's life was in jeopardy, I told them that there was nothing more that I could do and I waited outside for a while to let them be alone and talk things over. On my return, they were packing to go to the hospital.

The world of childbirth has come a long way in the past twenty years, for better and for worse. Instead of the alienation that fathers experienced in the earlier part of this century, an involvement in the process of birth has helped fathers to have a richer bonding experience with their newborn. They have been able to witness at first hand the hard work that the mother has had to perform as a result of the unification of the seed and the egg. I believe that birth needs to be a family affair. The touch of her husband's hand, a kiss, or just an encouraging word can give the mother the strength to continue on through one of the most challenging times in her life. Many men have expressed to me the deeper respect that they now have for their partners after watching their hard work. They have also expressed the helplessness that they feel during labor, wishing that they could share the "burden" of what their partners have to go through, but many have felt that they were able to do something just by being a support person. By being available for the laboring mother and being strong and calm, the father can give the mother strength and courage to go on.

As a midwife, I never want to take over the father's role at the time of labor. At times I have to hold myself back because when I see what needs to be done, it is sometimes quicker just to do it myself than to give instructions on what to do or how to do it. If I take on the father's role, however, I feel I am intruding. In a sense, this would be a form of intervention that could lead to problems for the family. This is the couple's birth; I am there only to give guidance, to monitor the mother and the baby, and to step in if an emergency situation arises. The father's involvement is important for the bonding of the family. Father, mother, and baby are working as a team to accomplish the miracle of life. If the father is not involved, a void may be felt. However, I am not promoting that the couple should attempt a birth alone. They do need an experienced birth attendant to assist and guide them, and that is where I come in.

What does the father's involvement entail while his wife is working to get the baby out? It is simple: just loving her and looking after her needs; rubbing her back, getting a cold glass of water and a cold cloth, and wiping her forehead; reminding her that all this work is to have a baby and how much he loves her for doing all this work. I always tell the dads that it is their job to remind the mother to urinate every hour and to keep track of fluid intake. The fathers can be in the tank toward the latter half of the labor and snuggle up to the mother or support her while squatting. The only reason why I caution the dads not to get into the tank too early is to prevent the water from clouding up faster. Or, if the amniotic sac has ruptured, then the father getting into the water early on in labor may introduce yet more foreign bacteria. Frequently, all that the women in labor need is to have their partners close to them. I can remember one particular birth in which the father was so extremely nervous that all he could do was cook and clean up the kitchen after he cooked. He was a professional chef, so we had all this wonderful food to nibble on while we waited for the baby to come. However, he was never with his wife; he was always in the kitchen. When we would tell him to go to his wife, he made the excuse that either he had to clean up or he had something ready to come out of the oven. Well, after almost twenty-four hours of labor, he finally caught on and went to her side and held her hand. An hour of being close to him made all the difference; she shifted into strong labor and gave birth a few hours before dawn.

If the father is willing, I instruct him ahead of time on how to catch the baby. I will be close by while the child is being born so that I can monitor what is going on in case there is something that the father might miss due to inexperience. I feel his catching of the baby is a completion of the circle; he plants the seed and in turn he receives the fruit. The family unit is very holy and should not be disturbed at one of the most miraculous times in the family's life.

Whether your goal is to have your baby born in the water, or simply to labor in the water, water's qualities are a superb medium to facilitate a natural childbirth. I have never witnessed anything that is better for empowering a woman to relax, enabling her to use her intuitive abilities to give birth without drugs or other forms of intervention. Whether or not water has been used in past centuries for laboring or delivering, it is now being used in most parts of the world as a means of supporting women to labor in a natural way, to labor without harming themselves or their babies.

7

===

SECOND STAGE: PUSHING

When a woman in labor is told that it is time to push, a great relief sweeps over her. It is like the last stretch in the race for the long-distance runner. The finish line is in sight. Being able to push is a reward in itself. The hard-working mother knows that this is the last stretch, that with a little more work, she will hold in her arms the fruit of her labor. There is also the anticipation, especially from a first-time mother: How hard will pushing be? Will I be able to get my baby out? I don't know if I can go on any longer!

The pushing stage is quite different from the first stage. Contractions are now more dispersed and are spaced farther apart. They seem to be giving the mother a chance to rest and recharge, so that she will have the energy to push the baby out. I encourage the mother to sleep between contractions, to take advantage of the lulls that nature provides and recharge herself. The laboring mothers are so beautiful during these resting times, looking as if they were kissed by an angel. Anyone present can sense the room filled with the spirit of the forthcoming child.

The warmth of the water helps the mother to go into a deep, nourishing sleep. Some might call it a meditation. When the next contraction awakens her, she feels refreshed with more energy to push. I have observed that sleeping in water gives the person a deeper sleep than on a bed. It appears that the mothers awake with more strength and energy. After the contraction is finished, I remind the mother to take sips of water with some maple syrup or honey mixed in. This puts sugar in her system, giving her more energy to push.

In Chapter 6, I stated that the buoyancy of water helps the laboring mother to move more freely. During the pushing stage, the water helps the mother get into the various positions that she feels comfortable in and are necessary to get the baby out. Depending on the depth of water in the tank, several positions can be used to push the baby out. I encourage the mother to use her instincts as to what position is suitable for her.

Many believe that the supported squat is the best possible way to give birth, for several reasons:

1. Working with gravity helps pull the baby down and out.

2. This position allows the whole pelvic area to open up to its maximum capacity.

3. Since all areas of tissue have equal pressure, tearing is a smaller possibility.

4. The fetus receives the optimal amount of oxygen since there is less compression on the head and on the blood vessels that feed the uterus oxygen.

A deep tank is needed as the standing-supported squat in its true form raises the mother to a near standing position. Someone is behind her holding her up so that she may use all her strength to push. The water in the tank would have to be too deep for laboring in if the mother wanted to give birth into the water in a standing-supported squat. The only type of tank that seems to work is a spa that has built-in seats, allowing different water levels. I have seen a few couples give birth this way when using the spa.

By using a lower squat with or without someone behind her, a shallower tank can be used. The laboring mother may hold onto the sides of the tank or can be assisted by someone behind her. If a shallow tank such as a bathtub is used, a semisitting position will better facilitate the emergence of the baby into the water.

The hands and knees or elbows and knees position has worked in a tank that has a deeper level of water. In addition, the mother may put her arms around someone's shoulders and squat; hang onto a child's swim raft; or comfortably rest on a bench or ledge. Most likely the birthing mother will automatically get into whichever position feels best for her and whichever will better facilitate the birth of the baby.

I have found that the water in the tank should be no less than 18 inches, so that there is enough water to cover the woman's belly, and it should not rise much higher than the mother's breasts when she is sitting on the bottom of the tank. It should not be too deep primarily because the mother can become easily overheated. One mother said that when the water was up to her neck she felt claustrophobic and

Figure 4
The Supported Squat

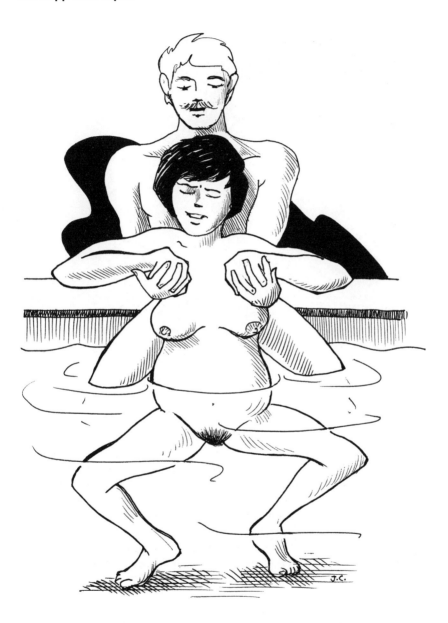

Figure by Jeff Cox

Figure 5
Squatting while Leaning against the Side of the Tank

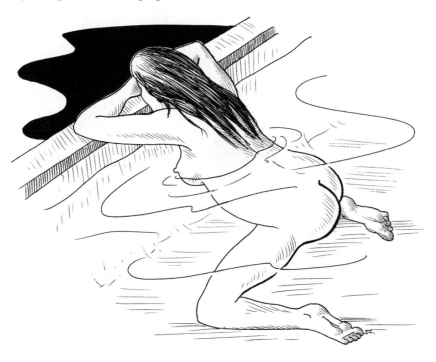

Figure by Jeff Cox

asked that some water be taken out. She also reported that it was harder to move about when the water was too deep.

The temperature of the water may vary during the pushing stage, depending on the comfort of the mother. Ideally, the temperature should be around 100° F when the baby is born, but the water can be cooler for the mother while she is pushing. Bringing the water temperature up quickly can be accomplished by turning the waterbed heaters up full blast or by having some big kettles of water heating on the stove to add to the water before the baby is born. *Be careful in adding the hot water so as not to scald the mother.* Add the water slowly and away from the area where the mother is and swirl it through the tank with your hand.

HOW PUSHING IN WATER DIFFERS

When comparing the traditional homebirth with an underwater birth, I have noticed that in some cases the pushing stage may be slowed down when the mother is in the water. In other words, in some cases, the baby does not advance through the birth canal as quickly as in a delivery that is out of the water. This may be attributed to the lesser force of gravity in the water pulling on the baby. Another theory is that because the mother is more relaxed, she feels less urgency about getting the baby out. The observations I have made regarding the slower advancement of the baby during the pushing stage needs further study. The contractions are as strong, but at times, progress is not made as quickly. The baby is making a slower movement, a slower progression.

Getting into a supported-squatting position, in or out of the water, may help to speed up the birth. At times getting out of the tank is a necessity if the pushing stage is taking too long and the mother is getting exhausted. Getting out of the tank and pushing are also necessary if the heart tones are wildly swinging, indicating that the baby is under stress. The baby then needs to come out as soon as possible. If the baby's heart tones have returned to a safe range and the baby's head has made good advancements and is starting to show, the mother may return to the tank to safely deliver the baby. As in the first stage, one may get in and out of the tank as desired or needed, remembering to rinse the feet in the betadine solution upon entering the tank.

The mother can work with gravity by walking around and squatting when a contraction comes on. Women can use their partners for a birthing chair by sitting on their partners' knees and pushing, and then sit back down in the water when the baby's head starts showing. Some women have found that sitting on the toilet can also act as a birthing chair. The mother can more easily get in touch with using the same muscles to push the baby out as those she uses in having a bowel movement. The midwife needs to be close at hand and to monitor the baby's progress so that the baby is not born in the toilet. If necessary, I will monitor the descent of the head with my two fingers inside the mother's vagina to see how quickly the head is coming and get the mother back in the tank before the head starts showing. Once a bit of the head is showing, it is advisable to stay in the birthing tank and keep pushing. This slowing of the second stage usually happens with first-time mothers or mothers with large babies (9 to 10+ pounds).

Frequently, too, there can be a very short, quick pushing stage. The mother may be so surrendered and open that the baby may just slide out with a few pushes. This may be more intense for the mother when the pushing stage happens so quickly. I remind the mother that the pain will not last long and that she needs to push through the pain. The baby's heartbeat needs to be monitored after every contraction and during every other contraction to make sure that the baby is doing well during a precipitous delivery.

A NOTE TO MIDWIVES

The birth attendant should not be surprised if the second stage is a bit different from what she has seen in the traditional homebirth setting. She needs to be well versed and informed on the similarities and differences of a water birth as compared to a birth in the traditional home setting.

During the second stage the birth attendant plays a very important role. For some mothers, the adjustment from the laboring to the pushing stage may be difficult. Transition can shake the mother up and put her off center. Many first-time mothers need instructions on how to push, while women who have had other children may need reminding. The birth attendant can be like an anchor for the mother, someone to help direct her through the many different aspects of childbirth, especially the pushing (second) stage where the birth attendant takes a more active role. Before the pushing stage begins, the birth attendant and the mother need to go over the breathing techniques and the times to push and not to push. This can be a team effort that, with planning, can prevent the tearing of the perineum and will help the mother to conserve energy while making the pushing efficient and productive. This type of pushing will be discussed later in the chapter.

Occasionally, the mother is afraid to push for fear that it will hurt her or the baby. Being sensitive to the woman's fears and being reassuring are both essential. She should be reminded that women have been giving birth for millions of years and that millions of women have done what she is about to do. In simplistic terms, our bodies are made to give birth to carry on the species.

The birth attendant should have attended several water births or at least be well educated on the subject. If the attendant comes with a lot of intellectual fears about water births, however, she can do more harm than good. Anyone who is present at the birth should have a deep understanding of the theories of water births, have read as much information as possible, and have seen some videos on water births. And, of course, voyeurs have no place at the birth. The only people who should be present are people with whom the mother feels comfortable and are there for help and support, not just to watch a baby being born. Many birth practitioners believe the fewer people at the birth the better. Too many people can distract the mother while laboring and can drain her energy.

DIFFERENT TYPES OF PUSHING

The breathing methods that can be the least wearing on the mother involve the following: wait until the contraction starts building, take a deep breath, then push on the exhalation during the height of the contraction. This method of pushing helps the mother become less exhausted. Pushing during the height of the contraction may make the pushing stage longer. In the case of big babies, more aggressive pushing is needed. It is effective and can further as much progress as the following methods.

When the previously mentioned method of pushing doesn't bring the baby down any lower, the birth attendant may need to instruct the mother to put all her energy into pushing, to push with the entire contraction, being cautious not to wear herself out and not to get dizzy.

When the contraction is coming on, take a deep cleansing breath and let it out. Take another deep breath and hold it. Put your chin down into your chest, and using the same muscles that one would use to have a bowel movement, then PUSH! After the contraction is over, take some deep breaths to get oxygen to oneself and the baby. If the mother desires a breath from the oxygen tank, this may be appropriate to ease the dizziness and to get some extra oxygen to the baby. Many women get dizzy and lightheaded when they push as hard as possible during the entire contraction. A breath of oxygen from the oxygen tank can help the mother with any lightheadedness and will bring some oxygen to the baby as well. Then rest.

As already noted, the contractions are not usually as close in the pushing stage as in the first stage, which gives the mother ample time to drift off and relax, preparing for the next contraction. This is also an opportune time to listen to the baby's heartbeat, whether in or out of the water. Again, depending on the progress made with the pushes, the woman may want to push with the entire contraction or at the height of the contraction. The midwife needs to give the mother feedback on whether or not the mother is pushing effectively. Sometimes it is hard to get in touch with what muscles to push and how to push. The midwife can work with the mother and instruct her as to how to do this if the mother finds pushing difficult.

Some women have difficulty with pushing, but with careful guidance the mother will soon become a pro at pushing her baby out. While not all women have the uncontrollable urge to push, others cannot stop themselves from pushing.

During the pushing the mother may push some feces out into the water. Someone should be in charge of the pooper scooper (the aquarium fishnet) and get the feces out as soon as possible. Since the enema is given during the first stage, usually just a small amount of feces is passed. This is no problem, but it should be dealt with immediately. It is usually one of the birth attendant's concerns. Will the feces in the water cause an infection in the mother or baby? By 1993, in many parts of the world, approximately four thousand babies had been born under water. To my knowledge no infections due to the water have ever been reported. Nonetheless, every precaution needs to be taken to ensure its cleanliness for both mother and baby.

When the baby's head is presenting on the perineum, it is time to stop pushing. Not pushing can be very difficult. It is easy to get "swallowed up" by the intensity of the birth process, losing one's focus on not pushing and getting lost in the pain and one's fears. Helping the mother to focus on someone's eyes and blowing as hard as possible will help prevent the mother from pushing. If there is little progression of the head showing at the perineum, the mother may need to give some little pushes, but she needs to stop when she can feel her perineum stinging. This is a signal that the perineum may be beginning to tear and the mother needs to start blowing (with pursed lips, as if blowing out a candle, only a lot harder), or panting (like a dog), to prevent herself from pushing. This breathing method forces the mother to think about something other than pushing. The uterus is an involuntary muscle and will push the baby out on its own. I have seen some women omit the voluntary pushing during the entire second stage, relying totally on the uterus to push the baby out, needing just a few extra pushes on the mother's part.

Sometimes this is efficient pushing, sometimes not. This nonaggressive pushing will be a lot slower, which may also slow the progress of the birth. If the baby's heartbeat is within the normal range, allowing the uterus to do the pushing may be fine. The nonaggressive pushing will minimalize the force of the push and (along with the blowing breath) prevent tearing of the perineum. The baby will then have a slower, less traumatic exit. However, if little progress is being made over one hour of pushing and the baby's heartbeat is getting erratic, then it may be time for the mother to start pushing more aggressively and possibly get out of the water.

PERINEAL MASSAGE

The perineal massage can help prevent the tearing of the perineum. This massage is performed in the same manner as in any childbirth, with the exception that oil on the perineum is omitted. Before the head starts crowning, the person catching the baby should start the perineal massage by putting light pressure on the floor of the vagina with the index and middle fingers. A sweeping motion is made from the bottom of the vagina to each side of the outer vagina, encouraging stretching and blood circulation. When the *top* of the head is entirely out (the crowning), the massaging should continue on the outside of the perineum as well as on the sides of the vulva (the vaginal lips). Supporting the perineum is important once the head starts slipping through. This can be accomplished by putting pressure against the perineum with the palm of one's hand while the head is coming through. The warmth of the water helps the tissues stretch well. Before I attended water births, I would apply warm compresses to the perineum during the pushing stage. The warmth and moisture of the water along with the perineal massage helps keep the tissues pink and the blood well circulated. If the perineal massage is part of the daily routine during pregnancy, then the tissue around the vaginal opening is used to stretching.

When water births were first introduced in the United States, people believed that if the mother gave birth in the water she would automatically be predisposed to an intact perineum. Theoretically, this may sound logical because of the warmth of the water. However, it should not be used as an excuse to slack off on the preparatory perineal massage during the pregnancy. No one can predict how quickly the baby will emerge from the vaginal opening. He may emerge with such force that there may be a tear, water birth or no. Large babies in a primapara mother (first-time mother) may also cause a tear. In my practice I have experienced mothers tearing. There is a lower incidence of it, however, with the warmth of the water, good perineal support, and the good teamwork of mother and midwife. It is important that no one set themselves up for disappointments. If preventing a tear is one of your main reasons for having a water birth, please remember that nature is not predictable and that there is a possibility of tearing all the same.

EPISIOTOMY

I have never done an episiotomy in the water, but I have talked to a few midwives who have. (An episiotomy is the cutting of the skin that is between the vaginal opening and the anus, to make a bigger opening for the baby to come out.) The midwives have said that the blood from the episiotomy can darken the water to the point where it is impossible to see the baby's face when born. If this is the case, then the baby should not be born into the water. A baby should never be born into water that is so clouded that his or her face cannot be observed. One couple told me that during their first water birth the midwife did the episiotomy above the water, letting the blood drip into a bowl; then the mother quickly squatted down in the water and gave birth. Most midwives do not routinely do episiotomies and will perform them only when absolutely necessary.

MONITORING THE BABY'S HEARTBEAT

Monitoring the baby's heartbeat during the pushing stage is essential. It is important to stay on top of things so that one can be alerted as to any stress that may occur in the baby. It is even more essential for a water birth. It is almost impossible to detect meconium in the water of the birthing tank if the bag of waters should rupture while the mother is in the water, even meconium that is the consistency of pea soup. I have been able to detect it at times, but only because I checked the mother soon after the waters broke, unaware that there had been a rupture. If complications arise, the mother may need to get out of the water and onto the bed that is beside the tank to deliver. With this in mind, I like to listen to the fetal heart tones (FHTs) after every contraction during the pushing stage, especially if the FHT starts swinging out of the normal range of 120 to 160 beats per minute. Checking after every contraction is a sure way of making sure the baby is doing well and can be safely birthed into the water. I also like to listen to the FHT during the contraction to assess how the baby is reacting to the stress of the contraction. I like to do this after every three or four contractions. The FHT may become ten to fifteen beats faster during the contraction, but will get back to the previous range prior to the contraction.

As I stated earlier, several different pieces of equipment can be used to monitor the baby's heartbeat. I prefer to use a doppler with a remote lead, such as the Parks doppler. The remote lead can be immersed in the water. This way the FHT can be listened to more quickly and more easily. Raising the mother's hips out of the water to get at the abdominal region can be uncomfortable for the mother but may need to be done depending on what type of equipment is being used. If using a fetoscope or a doppler that is all one unit, the mother will have to get out of the water or else lift her hips out of the water. The Parks remote lead can be immersed in the water and can be accessible to the mother no matter what position she is in.

Another advantage of using a doppler in a water birth is at the point where the fetal heart tones pass behind the symphysis pubis. The heart tones can be hard to find or may get lost entirely. Losing the FHT can be crucial at any birth. Guess work is not appropriate, especially if the FHTs have been swinging dramatically. It is necessary to keep on top of the monitoring at a water birth, making sure that it is appropriate to continue in the water.

Being in the tank while the child is being born has been very essential for me. I have felt estranged from the birth if I am alongside the tank with only my hands in the water. Water is an excellent conductor for sound and electricity. Igor Charkowsky feels it is also a strong conductor of psychic energies, possibly transmitting the feelings of the baby, if there are problems arising with the mother. Therefore, being in the water helps the midwife become part of the birth process with mother and baby. If the tank is not big enough for me to get in along with the father and mother, I'll stay along the side and watch and assist the birth.

At the Pre- and Perinatal Psychology Conference in 1987, where I was speaking on water births, a European doctor asked me how I protect myself from AIDS while attending a water birth. I ask both mother and father to have an HIV test during the last month of the pregnancy. In addition, during the initial screening, I find out if either of them has had any blood transfusions or is an intravenous drug user. I'll be so bold as to take the father and mother aside separately and ask if they are having extramarital sex. I personally will not attend a water birth with someone who is HIV positive. It is too risky for all those involved, especially since the baby may need extra medical attention at the birth. I have met midwives who feel comfortable doing homebirths for women who are HIV positive, but not in the water.

THE FATHER'S INVOLVEMENT IN THE SECOND STAGE

Using my intuition is one of the key tools of my art as a birth attendant. Another important aspect of my work is knowing when to keep out of the picture and become the proverbial fly on the wall. Stepping aside and letting the mother and father participate as much as possible in the procedures to help birth the baby can be one of the more empowering episodes in both the mother's and father's life. I purposely involve myself only when the couples need guidance, assistance, or emergency attention. I will step in and give my advice if I see a possible emergency arising which could be prevented by taking certain steps.

Women need to take the power of birth into their own hands, not to give it away. Finding that strength, finding that center of power, can transform a woman, enabling her to proceed through life with more strength and any of life's obstacles that may occur. In addition, the father's involvement with the catching of the baby is important for him. It makes him feel more involved, for now he is a real part of the birthing process. I like to coach the father through the delivery, having my hands on as well. Unless a person is experienced, I will do little things such as checking to see if the cord is wrapped around the neck. It is also necessary to determine whether there is a pulse in the cord. With this involvement, he and the mother work as a solid team, making decisions and sharing in the miracle of life. I coach the father during the pregnancy on how to do the perineal massage, and I encourage him to read the midwifery books on how to catch the baby. He should also be well versed in what complications can occur as well as in how to deal with them, so that he can make an informed decision on what steps to take in case of an emergency and why they need to be taken. The midwife should be at his side guiding and rechecking when the delivery is imminent. This can be done in a very nonintrusive way so that the father can be the person catching the baby, while the midwife is taking the safety precautions and monitoring.

THE EMERGENCE OF THE BABY INTO THE WATER

The baby's head will slowly start emerging. At first, a small part of the top of the head will be showing. Once the baby's head is visible, it will advance and recede as it does in any birth. At this point, as long as things are going smoothly, the water birth is treated the same as any birth; there is little difference. The mother needs to keep her focus, and the father or midwife should be doing the perineal massage and helping her breathe and push. Then more and more head shows until the crowning, the point where the whole top of the baby's head is showing. The rest of the head will emerge soon after. While the rest of the head is emerging, the midwife or the father will do the perineal massage and give support to the perineum, while the mother blows instead of pushing. When the head of the baby is born, I like to take the mother's hand and touch the baby's head, reminding her what all this work has been for.

Once the head is born, the midwife or father needs to slip two fingers along the side of the baby's head and into the mother's vagina to check if the cord is around the neck. The cord needs to be checked to see if it is strongly pulsing. As in any birth when the cord is wrapped around the neck, it is important to see if it is tight for it could strangle the baby or cut off the oxygen supply coming from the placenta. If it isn't, the mother needs to stand up and deliver the baby so that the baby may get oxygen as soon as possible. This is also true if the cord is tight around the neck. If the cord is too tight and needs to be cut with a blunt-nosed scissors (blunt nosed because regular scissors could puncture the baby), I ask the mother to stand up out of the water with someone supporting her, and I will cut the cord, freeing up the baby to move. With this procedure, the baby will be born into the air. If the cord feels loose enough that it can be unlooped, I will ask the mother to give a little push and unwrap the cord as the baby is emerging into the water. All those present should relax and enjoy, while the midwife monitors the baby's heartbeat by placing her fingers directly over the left nipple. The heartbeats should be in the same range as they were while the baby was in utero.

The head is usually born face down and will soon rotate to the right or to the left. This allows the shoulders to come out gracefully, and with another turn, the rest of the body will be born with the baby facing up. Check to see how the baby is doing by assessing the color of the baby's face and the sucking reflex. When I put my finger in the baby's mouth, the baby gives a little suck. I have seen the baby's face turn purple when it is out and the rest of the body is still inside the mother. This usually happens when the baby's head is sitting outside the vagina for one or two minutes. This tells me that it is time for the baby to come out and get into the air. The mother needs to give a strong push and deliver the rest of the body, possibly getting into the supported-squat position if the baby is not out quickly enough.

The midwife needs to watch for yet another signal while the head is out: Does the baby start making motions as if wanting to breathe? The mother should stand up and deliver the baby into the air. With most water births, I have seen the babies doing well with their heads out while waiting for the rest of their body to be born. I keep monitoring the fontanelle, watch the color of the baby, continue to check the cord, and watch for any signals that the baby may be making attempts to breathe. Occasionally, the body will make a slow emergence. This is all quite well, for it is thought that the slower the emergence, the less of an impact on the baby, and therefore the less trauma for the infant.

The body may slowly emerge to the chest and stay there for approximately thirty seconds to one minute. It is important to keep checking the fontanelle, as well as watching and monitoring the baby. The baby should show no signs of struggling or of making motions with the mouth as if gasping for air.

The baby may then emerge halfway out of the mother's body and again stop. I am a bit hesitant to allow the baby to stay there too long, not knowing whether or not the umbilical cord is being compressed against the symphysis pubis, thus cutting off blood and oxygen. If the baby does not move within a matter of seconds, I will ask the mother to give a gentle push, which totally frees the baby into the water.

HOW LONG DOES THE BABY STAY UNDER WATER?

One of the most frequently asked questions is, How long does one leave the baby under water? When underwater births first started becoming known in the early 1980s a few couples were leaving their babies under for fifteen to twenty minutes. Such a long period of time is not necessary and, in fact, is extremely dangerous. It is important at this point to set aside one's ego, to remember, as throughout the labor and delivery, what the main objectives and priorities are. Above all, we are not attempting any underwater marathons, nor are we attempting to set records for underwater durations. A minute or two under the water is the most that can be safe as long as close attention is paid to the baby. The parents and the birth attendant should agree beforehand on what guidelines to follow. Bringing the baby's face up immediately and leaving the body in the water will alleviate any concerns about the newborn inhaling water.

The important signs to pay attention to are: When unsubstantiated fears are set aside, what are your senses telling you? What are your gut-level feelings? Should the baby come up immediately? I usually leave this decision to the parents, but if I sense anything amiss, I will make the decision to bring the baby's face to the surface.

At the first four water births that I attended, the parents opted to keep the babies under the water for eleven to fifteen minutes. A few months after these births, I heard news of a birth somewhere in Southern California where a couple had no one in attendance, just the birthing mother and father. For some bizarre reason, the couple kept the baby under the water for an hour. Of course, the baby died. After hearing of this tragedy, I no longer felt comfortable being a proponent for keeping babies under the water for long periods of time. I felt that if I was going to be an advocate for water births, that safe guidelines needed to be established. Thereafter, I advised couples that a few seconds to the maximum of two minutes would be adequate. When I first started attending water births, not many babies had been born in this manner. Water births were still in a very experimental stage. All the couples agreed that a shorter time was more appropriate, especially when they saw that the baby had a good transition time in the water, that the baby was peaceful, and that the stress of birth seemed to be alleviated.

In the early days of water birth, alleviating labor's stress from the baby was the reason why many people were having their babies born into water, as well as allowing the mother greater comfort while laboring in the water. We quickly realized that the shorter period under the water was just as soothing and relaxing as the longer period. Some couples did not feel comfortable with leaving their babies under the water at all and brought their babies to the surface immediately. Their faces were brought out of the water, while the rest of the body was allowed to be free in the water. The baby's head, neck, and shoulders can be supported by dad's or mom's hands. Some mothers want to bring the babies immediately to the breast, while others want to let their babies have some transition time in the water.

When the baby is born, I immediately check the color of the umbilical cord. If it is white and flaccid, I bring the baby to the surface immediately, for this is an indication that the placenta may have separated, and with no blood in the umbilical cord there is no blood carrying oxygen to the baby. What I want to see is a strong pulsing cord that has a purplish-blue color, which indicates a strong blood and oxygen supply. I quickly place my index and middle fingers on the cord to monitor the pulse rate. Once there is a variation (meaning when the pulse starts slowing down), this signals to me that the placenta may be separating from the wall of the uterus. Another signal for this separation will be a gush of blood from the mother's vagina.

Depending totally on the monitoring of the umbilical cord is not sufficient. Checking the baby's heartbeat over the left nipple is the most reliable way to determine the condition of the baby. The part of the cord that is closest to the baby does keep pulsating even after the placenta is born. I experienced this at a water birth where the placenta was birthed without the cord being cut. The placenta was born forty-five minutes after the baby was born, during which time the cord pulsed strongly and continued to do so fifteen minutes after the birth of the placenta. It is important to note at which end the cord is pulsing. When monitoring the cord, I put my fingers about one inch away from the vaginal opening so that I am feeling the pulse as close as possible to the placenta. Nowadays, I put less emphasis on the pulsation of the cord than I used to. Yet other factors outweigh the cord pulsations in determining when to bring the baby to the surface of the water. (I will discuss these factors throughout this chapter.)

At the second water birth that I attended, the baby was born with a cord that was completely flaccid; the cord was as thin as a shoe lace and completely white. I had been monitoring the FHT throughout the pushing stage, and the beats were definitely within safe parameters. I was surprised to see such a flaccid cord inasmuch as everything else appeared to be fine. The baby was born into the water very peacefully, with no signs of oxygen deprivation, and pinked up soon after we brought her out of the water, which, in total, was approximately twenty seconds after the delivery. The mother delivered the placenta about twenty-one minutes after the birth of the baby. We brought this baby to the surface immediately because of the lack of oxygen in the umbilical cord. There are no reasons to take any chances. If all does not seem well, do not leave the baby under the water even for a second.

Along with monitoring the cord, I still monitor the fontanelle, alternating this with placing two fingers over the left nipple of the baby to check on the heartbeat. If the FHT drops below 110, which is beyond my safety parameters, I bring the baby to the surface.

Together with intuiting what the baby is feeling, there are certain physical signs to be aware of. Babies born underwater are not the typical tense, crying, tight-fisted little ones that we see in the hospital or even the traditional homebirth setting. They appear to be asleep, peaceful, and content. It is as if they are still in the womb, having forgotten about the labor and not knowing that they have been born.

Because the baby is still dependent on the umbilical cord and has not had the environmental stimulus to start breathing on his own, he will not have the typical newborn coloring. In a nonaquatic setting, one looks for a pink baby with perhaps a bluing in the extremities. This should not be expected in a water baby, although I have seen babies born in the water that are pink. The color of the infant will seem pale to blue. If the baby is a dusky color, a reassessment of the baby's condition may be in order; that is, check heart tones and umbilical cord, and look for a discharge of blood from the mother's vagina, signaling the release of the placenta. This dusky color may not be healthy and could mean that the baby is having problems adjusting to extrauterine life. Use your judgment. Bringing the baby to the surface may be necessary.

The midwife should also monitor the newborn's muscle tone. The water baby may not have the tenseness or tightness that is common in newborns, but will have muscle tone and response. Many of the water babies I have attended will lie quietly in a supported float, with possibly some kicking and movement of arms. There is also a reaction when I stroke the sole of the infant's foot. This is the Babinski reflex, and the toes will fan out as in any other birth setting. When I put my finger in the palm of the newborn water baby, the baby often will take hold of the finger. If I am still questioning the newborn's condition, I will put my finger in the baby's mouth to see if the baby has the sucking reflex. One concerned midwife gently put her little finger a little way into the baby's anus, which tightened up as it should with any healthy baby.

Once the baby has been brought from the water, it is beneficial for him to be placed in the crook of either the father or mother's arm, on his stomach, with his head lowered down so that any mucus that is in the oropharynx can drain out.

Water babies appear to be very serene or not awake. Some postulate that because of the gentle transition from the womb to the water, the soul/spirit is not quite shocked into total physical awareness. Often the comment that is made is, "The little one doesn't know he is born." To reiterate, this dormancy is fine as long as all the signs that I have discussed are apparent and the baby is functioning well. On a rare occasion, the baby does not like being under the water. This becomes apparent when the baby makes grimacing faces or appears to be restless. I have seen two babies make facial expressions as though they were crying. This can be attributed to a stressful birth. I have brought these babies to the surface immediately, concerned that they may have inhaled water. Upon suctioning them with a bulb syringe, there was no sign of any water aspiration in either mouth or nostrils. Their lungs also sounded clear when I listened to them with a stethoscope. I still feel that I made the right move by bringing them to the surface.

The midwife needs to assess things carefully. I have watched babies who, due to the stress of the birth, appear to be stressed for a minute or less. I watch to see if the water is relieving the stress or adding to it. After about one minute, if the baby is not showing signs of any relief while in the water, he needs to be brought up. A baby who is obviously unfolding and relaxing may stay in a bit longer.

How long may the baby stay under water if all conditions are favorable? First, use good judgment; proceed with caution and enjoy the beauty that is unfolding before you. In my experience, the average length of time may be approximately two minutes. Within this period the baby has a chance to feel the freedom of going from a smaller pool—the womb—to a place where he can rest—the warm water in the tank—while making the transition from womb to world. I personally have attended few births where babies are as totally at peace as they are in the water.

The peacefulness of the baby in the water gives us a glimpse of life in utero, as if we were looking through a window placed in the mother's belly. The peacefulness feels holy, evoking for every person in the room the warmth of the miracle that has occurred. One cannot help but feel the stillness and timelessness. Birth can be beautiful and simple, need not be complicated and chaotic. Yes, we are dealing with the fine string that connects both life and death. It is not to be taken lightly. The transition from womb to life is to be treated ever so delicately. The water enhances the birth experience for mother and baby. I have seen beautiful homebirths executed in the comfort of the family bed, but not as often as I have witnessed in the births of those born in the water. Those who fear water births may simply fear the unknown. No one should be flippant and cast fate to the wind at any time during any birth, but by taking precautions and listening to intuition, a beautiful water birth can be achieved. To my knowledge, of the approximately four thousand water births around the world, only two deaths have been recorded. The deaths were due not to the water itself, but to the parents' failure to have a skilled childbirth attendant at their birth. This is a better average than most hospitals have.

THE DELIVERY OF THE PLACENTA, OR THIRD-STAGE LABOR

Another frequently asked question is: Does the mother give birth to the placenta in the water? As with the pushing stage, delivery of the placenta—the third stage of labor—may take longer due to laboring in the water. In a traditional birth setting, the placenta will follow approximately twenty minutes after the birth of the baby. In the case of water births, I have found that the length of time for delivery is approximately forty-five minutes, and the maximum, an hour. After the birth of the baby, usually fifteen to twenty-five minutes, the mother feels ready to get out of the tank. Often, women express a sense of completion after the baby is born and brought out of the water. They feel no reason to stay in the tank any longer and may want to lie down on the bed. This is one reason why mothers deliver the placenta out of the water. Along with the mother being tired, it can be difficult to estimate blood loss while she is in the water. One cup can appear to be two quarts when mixed with water. As I have learned through experience, estimating blood loss is a bit tricky.

While the mother is still in the tank and the placenta is still attached, I am constantly monitoring her to see if any bleeding is occurring. In particular, I watch to see how quickly the water gets red and how dark it gets. The placenta may be separating itself from the wall of the uterus before one expects. As in any delivery, the midwife needs to watch the mother's face for any signs that she is not doing well. Is she getting pale or drifting off? Checking to make sure that the height of the fundus (top of the uterus) is staying below the mother's navel will help to determine whether or not to aggressively hasten the delivery of the placenta by squatting and pushing, or simply to wait longer for the placenta than is customary. Watching for contractions and the rising of the top of the uterus helps to distinguish whether or not the mother may be bleeding internally with the placenta still inside. If the fundus starts rising over the top of the mother's navel, this condition could indicate that the mother is bleeding internally. The mother then needs to get out of the water and deliver the placenta either lying down or squatting. The placenta may be birthed into a large bowl or onto a chux (blue pad) that is placed underneath her.

It is sometimes easy to get sidetracked by the newborn, and not pay enough attention to the mother. One birth in particular comes to mind. Everyone was oohing and aahing over the beautiful new baby, when someone noticed a small stream of blood coming from behind the mother. The midwife had her get out of the water immediately and began working on getting the placenta out. Fortunately, the placenta came soon after with little blood loss. As noted earlier, estimating the mother's blood loss is the trickiest part of a water birth. Although I have had no problems with hemorrhaging, I encourage the mother to pay close attention to any contractions she may be having. I remind her that the contractions for the placenta are not going to be as strong-feeling as those that she had to push the baby out. I also remind her that sometimes these contractions are easy to miss and that the mother does not get many of them.

It is wonderful to see the baby go to the breast with the mother still in the water. If the mother is watched carefully, she can safely nurse while in the water. When the blood starts trickling out of the mother's vagina, however, I feel that it is time to get the mother and baby out.

One father had an interesting suggestion for instructing professionals with regard to estimating blood loss. He said to go to a stockyard and purchase some blood; pour measured amounts of blood into the tankful of water and get familiar with the color of the water. Then, he said, see how quickly it reaches the darker colors with the amount of blood that you are using.

While in the former Soviet Union, working with Charkowsky, I was shown films of Russian women giving birth to the placenta in the water with no problems. There was not much blood loss, and they suffered no water embolisms. One concern here is that if the mother gives birth to the placenta in the water, that water will get into the uterine sinuses once the placenta has left the site open, travel through the blood stream to the lungs or heart, and kill the mother. This may be a consideration, but mostly I feel uncomfortable with women delivering the placentas into the water because of the problem of estimating blood loss.

For the sake of clarity, an explanation of an embolism is necessary. For example, Arthur Guyton's *Textbook of Medical Physiology* (1976) describes an embolism as an abnormal blood clot in the vessel that breaks away from its site of attachment and starts flowing freely. The text states that the embolisms originated in the large arteries or in the left side of the heart, eventually plugging smaller arteries or arterioles. The embolisms that originate in the veins or the right side of the heart will flow into the vessels of the lungs and cause a pulmonary embolism. *Williams Obstetrics* (Hellman, 1971) discusses an amniotic fluid embolism that brings the scenario closer to how a water embolism could occur. The book states that an amniotic fluid embolism is due to a very rapid labor and may accompany a rupture of the uterus. The amniotic fluid may go into the open venous sinuses of the placental site as well as the endocervical vein and then enter the general circulation, eventually going into the pulmonary veins. The fear is that the water may enter the same way as the amniotic fluid would through the open uterine sinuses and travel through the blood into the lungs, eventually causing death.

To my knowledge, no water embolisms have ever occurred during any water births. Since water births were first introduced in this country, water embolisms have been a major concern of the medical establishment questioning the safety of giving birth into water. While attending the First International Water Birth Conference in Tutukaka, New Zealand, I brought up the question of water embolisms before a panel of obstetricians and midwives. Air embolisms and amniotic fluid embolisms, I was told, are extremely rare, yet amniotic fluid embolisms occasionally occur in women who have very quick labors; in situations where the placenta detaches itself from the wall of the uterus before the baby is born (placenta abruptio); in rupture of the uterus; and in women who have precipitous labors after administration of pitocin or oxytocin. An Australian obstetrician told me that the only time he had seen a vaginal water embolism was during a waterskiing incident where the woman, after attempting a jump, landed with such great force that water was forced up into her vagina. Back in the states, another obstetrician informed me that the only time he had seen an air embolism was when a gentleman blew air from his mouth hard into his lady friend's vagina, causing an air embolism. As of 1993, no water embolisms due to birthing in the water had been recorded anywhere in the world.

All of these concerns can be alleviated by simply giving birth to the placenta out of the water. After the baby is born, the mother needs to be reminded to watch for another coming contraction. This contraction will be the one that will give birth to the placenta, and it will not be as strong as the pushing contraction, making it easier to miss. By the time this contraction arrives, the mother has usually gotten out of the tank and can give birth to the placenta where she pleases. If the time is coming on to an hour and the placenta has not yet come, I have a bowl placed in the toilet basin and let the mother sit on the toilet; gravity will aid in the delivery of the placenta. Remember, the placenta may take longer to be born in a water birth than a traditional home birth. I have had no problem with forty-five minutes to an hour, as long as someone is watching to make sure that the fundus does not reach the mother's navel.

In my mind the birth is not over until three hours after the delivery of the placenta, when any excess bleeding has returned to normal, when the baby is functioning well on her own, and mother and baby are tucked safely into bed.

APGAR SCORING

Typically, Apgar scoring was designed for hospital births where tests are made on the newborn at one minute after birth and again at five minutes after birth to assess how the newborn is adapting to extra-uterine life. Apgar scoring is based on five signs ranked in order of importance and a scoring of 0–10.

	0	**1**	**2**
Color	blue/pale	body pink, limbs blue	completely pink
Respiratory Effort	absent	slow, irregular weak cry	strong cry
Heart Rate	absent	slow, less than 100	over 100

Muscle Tone	limp	some flexion of limbs	active movement
Response to Flicking Foot	absent	facial grimace	crying

All these points are added up in their different categories to give the total score. A healthy Apgar score at one minute is 7 or 8 and at five minutes 9 or 10. Adding up the Apgar scores gives you an idea of how the baby is doing at the two different intervals. If the baby's heart is slow (below 100 BPM) and there is little detectable breathing, start CPR and get an emergency team on the way.

Apgar scoring at homebirths is slightly different from that in the hospital. It is done less aggressively, and so, too, is the scoring at a water birth. When doing the Apgar score for a water baby, the first minute is done while under the water, if the parents decide that they want the baby under. I score in the same way as one would at any birth for the heartbeat. The muscle tone is adequate if there is a response to the Babinski reflex or to any other muscle stimulation. The baby's color is usually pale at a water birth, because the carbon dioxide/oxygen exchange has not yet kicked in (although I have seen some pretty pink babies born into the water). If a baby has a dusky or bluish-purplish color, the baby should be brought to the surface immediately. All the five categories for an Apgar score can be used except, of course, the respiratory efforts at the first minute. At five minutes, all five categories can be assessed, for the baby should not be under the water. If the heart rate is 100 or under, bring the baby to the surface. The heart can usually be monitored accurately by placing two fingers over the left nipple. There is no difference in the heartbeat of a baby born in or out of water.

The baby should not be making any respiratory efforts under the water. Bring the baby to the surface if this should occur.

After about fifteen to twenty seconds, when the baby is out of the water, he should have taken his first breath. He may give a little sneeze or a snuffle and start crying or breathing. Often water babies do not cry and are very peaceful when born. If the baby is quiet and appears to be sleeping, watch for breathing movements. If these movements are not apparent within fifteen seconds, start massaging the spine upward, from the base of the spine to the base of the skull. Keep this up until the baby takes his breath or gives a cry. It seems that the babies do not know that they are born and are now independent souls. The massaging of the spine seems to awaken them, bringing them into their bodies.

The muscle tone of water babies will not be as tight since they are very relaxed when born. I have seen water babies lifting their hands out of the water or a foot out of the water, making movements that look like they are swimming. These are the same movements they make while in utero. When I move an arm or a hand, there is resistance, and the baby will move the arm back to where it was or to another place. This action demonstrates that the baby has muscle tone, that the baby is doing fine and is responding to stimuli. It is just important to remember that a tight-fisted, grimacing baby is not the norm for a water birth.

When I stroke the bottom of the water baby's foot, the foot normally reacts. I also find that if I put my finger in the baby's hand, he will react by holding the finger.

While the baby is still beneath the water, I do the first-minute Apgar scoring for the baby based on color, heart rate, muscle tone, and response to stimuli. The five-minute scoring is done as it usually is on a five-minute old newborn. (First minute means one minute after the baby is totally out of the mother; five minutes means five minutes after the baby is totally out of the mother.)

IMMEDIATELY AFTER THE BIRTH

A bulb syringe can be used very gently in the nose and the mouth to suction out the mucus. There is usually no water in the air passages. I have seen babies turn their faces to the side and take in some water as if to take a drink and let the water back out again. Occasionally, you can see the lung fluid being expelled from the baby while under water that looks like an opaque cloud. Michel Odent has an excellent photo depicting this phenomenon.

While in the Soviet Union I witnessed some births in which the mother did not use the bulb syringe to suction out the remaining mucus, but simply used her mouth. She placed her mouth over the nose and mouth of the newborn as if she were going to administer CPR, but instead sucked any mucus out that was left in the air passages. I like this method. It seems far less intrusive and just as efficient, using human contact instead of a foreign, hard rubber object. At times, getting the mucus out may be more difficult, and the bulb syringe may be necessary.

After things have settled down and the baby and mother are snug in bed, if it is appropriate (in other words if I am not disturbing the family bonding time) I will do the newborn exam and check the mother for tears, along with massaging her uterus to keep it toned. The midwife should also assess the placenta to make sure no pieces have been retained and also check the amount of blood the mother has lost.

Theoretically, once the baby has been brought to the surface, it may not be wise for the him to go back under the water, because he is no longer dependent on the umbilical cord for oxygen. His lungs are functioning, and he is breathing on his own. In all the excitement of the birth, the mother or father may accidentally let the baby slip under the water for an instant. Catching themselves, they bring the baby to the surface, with no harm done to the baby. Do not fear if this happens; the baby may sputter or cry and can be calmed. All the same, check and make sure that the baby is all right. Usually, what the baby needs is a little comfort and a chance to voice his opinion: "Get with it, mom and dad, and watch what you are doing!"

Charkowsky, a proponent of infant swimming, sees no problem in dunking the baby under the water soon after she is born. In fact, it is part of his program with water birthing. Soon after the umbilical cord is cut, Charkowsky starts dipping the baby under the water to get it used to swimming. He claims that we are all born with a breath-hold reflex and will lose this reflex if we do not continue water training. Many of the couples I have worked with have continued water training to some degree, working carefully with the infant and not holding him under for more than ten seconds.

Rн NEGATIVE WOMEN

For Rh negative women, cord blood and maternal blood can be taken after the birth, as in any birth at home or hospital. Speak with your midwife about your blood type to find out if the Rh factor is a concern. I prefer to do this once the mother and baby are in bed, simply because it is more convenient to take the blood from the mother and baby and give the RhoGAM shot to the mother.

Some voice concerns for babies being born into the water. Why doesn't the baby breathe under the water? One of the questions I tried to answer while doing research at the Stanford Medical Library was, What initiates the baby to take her first breath? I found that many theories have been proposed, none of them conclusive. Of particular interest to me in this respect was a paper by Abner Levkoff in which he confirmed what Charkowsky, Odent, and I had experienced:

> Several kinds of stimuli appear to operate simultaneously to evoke this initial extrauterine respiratory response. Biochemically, hypoxia, hypercapnia, and acidosis may all play a role in producing gasping, as they do in the fetus. *Perhaps of more importance in the nondepressed neonate are the thermal and tactile sensory impulses provoked by exposure to an extrauterine environment.* . . . It seems reasonable that neurally transmitted impulses which are independent of blood chemistry changes are especially important. When the neonate is born unimpaired, the pulmo-

nary transitions . . . take place smoothly within the first several minutes, at which time the infant is breathing with little, if any, visible retractions or grunting (emphasis added) (1982, p. 107).

Environmental factors such as change in temperature, gravitational pressure, sensory changes from intrauterine to extrauterine life, and air, along with placental separation, apparently play a big part in the baby taking the first breath. As long as all the precautions I have discussed in this chapter are taken and the midwife and the parents are in agreement, having a water birth should be a good experience for all involved, including the baby, who will not start breathing until brought up into the air within a safe time after birth.

THE IMPORTANCE OF A GENTLE BIRTH

Dr. Ruth D. Rice, who holds a Ph.D. in early child development and psychology, states in the *Journal of Neonatal Nursing* that

a stressful intrauterine environment, a traumatic birth, early separation of mother and infant, hospital environment where pain and stress are imposed on the infant, causing the "inhibition of action" [passive reaction to pain and body intrusions; no crying, no resistance] syndrome, and the deprivation of loving touch and body stimulation continuing through childhood can predispose the infant to a violent and aggressive personality. Every experience the human organism has is imprinted on the memory system in cortical cells and will be evidenced . . . during the life span of the individual (1985, p. 40).

Dr. Rice also writes about persons who have gone through age regression, reexperiencing their births. She believes that people can relive the birth trauma with great clarity and accuracy. When brought back to their birth, there is always the expression of anger, resentment, fear, pain, and a feeling of abandonment, she says. A two-year study conducted in 1982 by the California Commission on Crime Control and Violence Prevention stated that a positive, gentle, loving, and nontraumatic birth experience increases the likelihood of healthy child development and less violent behavior.

There is much evidence that confirms that birth leaves a lasting imprint on the newborn and on the mother as well. Many studies by various psychologists, doctors, midwives, and laypersons could be quoted to support the idea that a gentle, loving entry into the world is an extremely significant, if not the most significant impression that is ever made on a human being. We are cradled within the safety of our mother's womb. We are raw, open, and innocent, cognizant of every little movement and every little detail of our new extrauterine world. To welcome the new ones, there is water, a gentle, soothing, caressing, familiar environment that provides a place of nurturance and safety. Labor and birth in the water promote the finest entrance into this new world called life that a child can experience.

COMPLICATIONS IN THE WATER

Recently, I interviewed Betty, a nurse-midwife from California who has attended approximately 450 homebirths and a thousand hospital births. During her twelve years of experience as a midwife, she has attended twenty water births. She reports attending two separate water births where the babies seem to have made respiratory efforts while under water. She also claims to practice conservatively, not allowing the babies to stay under the water for more than thirty seconds. Both were very straightforward births. There were no decelerations in the babies' heartbeats in either birth and no meconium. One birth was very fast, and in this particular one she saw bubbles coming from the baby's mouth. The baby expelled water from his mouth, and more was taken out with a bulb syringe. The baby was breathing a bit shallow and the heartbeat was good, but did not respond immediately to stimuli. All was fine after a few minutes. The other baby who made the respiratory efforts had no problems but did take some water in the mouth. The nurse-midwife says that she still feels good about water births. "The benefits for both mother and baby far outweigh the low risk," she says. She also says she will continue to support women who want to have water births.

One complication that I have had to deal with a few times during a water birth is shoulder dystocia, or stuck shoulders. This occurs when the head of the baby is out of the mother's vagina and the shoulders are still inside, unable to move. If minutes pass and I cannot get the baby out, I will ask the mother to stand up out of the water and get into the standing-supported squat position. This position usually enables the baby to pass through; if not the position, then the movement itself does the trick. I sometimes get the mother into a hands and knees position, but I find that the squat works better to get the baby out. I don't feel comfortable delivering a baby with shoulder dystocia into the water, because the baby may need to get air immediately.

One evening at the Black Sea in the Crimea, Charkowsky and I discussed water births that were out of the ordinary. He claimed that breech babies were better off born in the water, since the warmth of the water was a similar environment to the warm amniotic fluid in the womb. One of the controversies about birthing breech babies vaginally is that cold air may hit the baby's body before the head comes out and could make the baby gasp and therefore inhale the amniotic fluid in the vagina. This is why warm towels are always wrapped around a breech baby when born vaginally. If the baby is in a complete breech positon (a position where the baby's buttocks are presenting first, rather than a footling where the legs are presenting first), it is safe to proceed with a water birth. As noted, it seems to Charkowsky that it would be even better for a breech baby to be born into the water. I told him that if this is so, then water births would be good for twins, since about 37 percent of the time one of the twins can be in a breech position. He seemed surprised by the comment, for birthing twins in the water did not seem at all unusual to him. I have not had the opportunity to work with twins in the water milieu, but I received a wonderful letter from Peggy, a midwife in Oregon who birthed her own twins in water. She tells her story in Chapter 9.

Water helps keep birth simple. Its nonobtrusive milieu creates an environment where there is no need for a pharmacological buffer, supporting the mother to be fully responsible and aware to give birth to a beautiful healthy baby.

8

==

POSTPARTUM

Trust yourself. You know more than you think you do. . . . It may surprise you to hear that the more people have studied different methods of bringing up children the more they have come to the conclusion that what good mothers and fathers instinctively feel like doing for their babies is usually best.

Benjamin Spock, quoted in Sally Emerson,
A Celebration of Babies

After the baby is born and the placenta is delivered, there is nothing more for the mother to do except to go to bed and enjoy her baby. The midwife can help her with the nursing if any problems arise, but usually mothers and babies can get right to it. It is not unusual for the baby not to nurse for a few hours. Occasionally, the baby will even go for a day without nursing. I always encourage my mothers to get in touch with their local La Leche League, which can be found in the telephone book. Almost every town has a chapter. La Leche League is a good support group that encourages breastfeeding, even when bottle feeding appears to be easier. I have never figured out how some women have concluded that bottle feeding is easier than breastfeeding—especially in the middle of the night. Nathaniel slept with me, and all I had to do was turn over and place the nipple in his mouth when he whimpered. It is so much easier than opening cans and placing the formula in the plastic bottle, then warming it. And look at the contents of the formula; if only babies could talk. . . .

It is wonderful for the family to get into bed together and be close right after the birth. I encourage the mother or father to put the naked baby on their bare breasts, so that the babies have good skin-to-skin contact. Babies love this and literally thrive on the closeness, the touching, and the love. This is especially important for little ones who have had traumatic births or been born prematurely.

If the mother would like to sleep and the baby has had her chance to nurse, then I encourage the father to have his bonding time with the baby. It is nice to take the baby back into the tank of warm water, unless the water has been badly soiled with blood and feces. This is the same principle as the Leboyer bath, but the baby has more room to stretch out and move.

Charkowsky gets the babies swimming immediately after birth. He feels the sooner the better, while the baby still has the breath-hold reflex and the swimming motions are still fresh in the baby's consciousness. I like to see the mother have her time with the newborn, and then the father can do the swimming. Some will gently float their babies around while others will start the instantaneous dunking to begin their baby's swim lessons.

The babies love it. They go into a deep relaxation and make the same movements they made while in utero. They will open their eyes, look at their daddies, and look around as if they are exploring their surroundings.

One newborn boy was happy only when he was in the water; he would cry when he was brought out. Even nursing did not seem to console him, so for about twelve hours we had to bring him in and out of the tank.

Many parents continue the water training. It is a fun activity to do with your child. During the first year, it gives the babies greater freedom of movement and stimulates the brain. Can you imagine just lying in bed all day on your back or your side? Then when you get a little older, you are able to be in a sitting position and that's it! While in the water, babies can move their arms and legs with a greater sense of freedom than when confined to land. Babies like to swim. Infant swimming introduces children to water that can become a lifetime enjoyment. I learned to swim babies through Igor Charkowsky and Claire Timmermans, the author of *How to Teach Your Baby to Swim* (1975). Remember the movie *The Blue Lagoon*? The beautiful baby swimming around in the lagoon was Timmermans'.

Many people ask me whether being born in the water makes a difference in how the child grows up. Are these children any smarter? Do they become less violent individuals? It is hard to say. Many impressions throughout the child's life can shape the way he or she behaves and thinks. I do believe that what the child perceives as he or she first comes into the world can leave a lasting impression, be it gentleness or violence. This impression is the looking glass through which the child will view the world. The likelihood of a healthy mind increases if the birth is gentle—and being born in water is gentle.

Parenting also leaves a lasting impression. Many of us have had traumatic childhoods whose effects have lingered into our adult lives, causing innumerable problems for us. Loving your child and giving good guidance are the basics for creating a healthy individual.

MOTHERING

> I recalled my psychology professor's explanation of why women are less productive than men. He had referred to a letter written by Harriet Beecher Stowe in which she said that she had in mind to write a novel about slavery, but the baby cried so much. It suddenly occurred to me that it would have been much more plausible if she had said "but the baby smiles so much." It is not that women have less impulse than men to be creative and productive. But through the ages having children, for women who wanted children, has been so satisfying that it has taken some special circumstance—spinsterhood, barrenness, or widowhood—to let women give their whole minds to other work (Margaret Mead, in Emerson, 1986, p. 76).

Being a mother transforms women. After birth, the mothering instinct blossoms, and priorities in life change, with beauty taking on new meaning. Motherhood may bring days of horrible depression and ecstatic elation beyond compare. The mood changes only reflect the hormones fluctuating; the hormones will eventually level out. The mother should relax and enjoy her baby, and if possible, stay in bed for the next two weeks and watch the miracle grow before her. Drinking two pots a day of a combination of red raspberry leaf tea and comfrey leaf tea is said to help heal and tone the uterus. The mother also needs to keep herself well hydrated by drinking plenty of water to help keep the milk flow going.

After a mother has given birth in water, she knows there is no other way. Women who have had babies prior to their first water labor and delivery say that there is no comparison. Water embraces the mother and says, "do it as only you know how." Water helps a mother to feel satisfied, complete, and whole, giving her the knowledge that she has given birth with love and respect for this new soul before her.

> A few hours after my son was born, I left our place of birth, our living room, and snuggled up in bed with him. It was early June. I awoke a few hours later to smell the soft warm rain. I looked at my baby beside me, blood of my blood, soul of my soul. The oak trees were peeping in through the windows at him. A robin sang her rain song. An overwhelming feeling of completion swept over me. I wept for joy (S. Napierala).

9

===

BIRTH STORIES

I recall the first water birth that I ever attended; it took place in the early 1980s. I had many questions that were still unanswered in my mind. I felt comfortable attending a water birth, but experience always speaks loudest, and previous to this water birth, I had no experience with birthing babies in water. After careful research, I came to the conclusion that water is safe for labor and delivery as long as precautions are taken. I also wanted to do my best, within reason, to support women in choosing whatever method they desired for giving birth.

The labor helped Rennie relax far more than in the previous labors where I had observed women using showers or bathtubs to relax. The pushing was even better; I didn't observe the hard straining that I observe in most women when they are in second-stage labor. Yes, Rennie had to work at pushing, but she said it was almost effortless in comparison to her first conventional homebirth.

When the baby's head first came out, I held my breath and momentarily examined my soul to see if I was doing the right thing in assisting this woman and man let their baby come into a medium that some considered harmful. I carefully watched little Robin slip out of her mother. How beautiful and delicate she was. She appeared to be asleep, unaffected by the process of birth, not knowing that she was born. Her face was serene. She didn't have the look of anguish of being tortured that so many newborns have at birth. Rennie remarked that Robin looked like Winnie the Pooh when Robin was half way out of her. At this point (half way out, half way in), Robin's eyes opened, she looked straight up into her dad's eyes, and slowly closed them, as if going back to sleep. Her arms were extended toward the top of the water. I put one of my fingers into the palm of her hand, and she gave the appropriate response: she held on to it. I began checking the heartbeat, which was within the normal range of a newborn. I checked the fontanelle for the appropriate number of beats. This, too, was good. After she had totally emerged from her mother, I checked her muscle tone, which was strong, and when I stimulated the bottom of her foot (Babinsky reflex), she responded appropriately by flaring her toes. As I stated earlier, screaming newborns with anguished faces are usually the norm for birth attendants. Not to see this look can be disconcerting, making birth attendants question whether or not the child is having trouble.

After Robin came to the surface, she took her first breath and sneezed. Robin was laid on her mother's breast to rest as she slowly learned to breathe on her own. She cooed instead of wailed. Listening to her lungs canceled out any fears of water aspiration. They sounded clear. Everyone in the room remarked how beautiful she was and questioned how anyone could believe that newborns are ugly. I reminded them that it isn't that the babies are ugly. The fact of the matter is that they have had such a difficult time with the birth and all the interventive procedures that have been imposed on them that anyone of us would look twisted and morose. Robin had an easy transition into this world, and her mother had an easier time during labor. Both factors account for the low amount of stress on the baby.

Michelle, a water birth mother from France, writes of her experience with a water birth:

There was a succession of painful contractions and relaxations. The midwife became very firm, not allowing me to drift off in my own universe; she recommended that I keep my eyes on my husband at my side by the tub and breathe deeply with him, which was hard. Crazy thoughts passed through my mind in those hellish times, like: "I darn wished I was a man and would not have to go through this" (a desire I had thought gone since adolescence) or "the hell with natural childbirth!," and I would emphatically declare to my husband this was the first and last time I would endure labor.

The dilation went pretty fast. I was surprised to learn I was in transition and that the pain was probably at its apex. When I heard I reached 9 cm, I sighed deeply and almost cried out of joy. I finally got the sign of pushing, and it was not difficult to practice it well. My midwife had me half-squatting on the toilet while she was refilling the bathtub and I made quicker progress there, though I missed the warm enveloping waters. I was glad I could use cool oxygen toward the end, for the room and water were quite hot for the coming of the baby, and I twice felt a little light-headed. The baby's heartbeat, after having started at 140 and dropping to 120 at the beginning of pushing, resumed a steady 130 until the end. The pushing time lasted about an hour, we think, though it's hard to say.

I felt so involved in the process all the time. (What's the story about watching the pain from the ceiling, not considering the contractions "painful" but "intense" and welcoming them?) I was so taken by it all that the night went by very quickly.

When I reentered the bathtub, my midwife warned me to follow her directions to avoid tearing. While pushing, I was holding my breath, but when I would start feeling a burning sensation at the perineum, I would pant to stop the pushing. I quickly learned to do this, and it felt good to exercise some kind of control now! I even felt some pleasure among the pain. It was not as bad as before. I felt very strong and remembered to keep opening while pushing. It's certainly a strange sensation, this big bowel-like movement!

The midwife got in the tub to press on my perineum as the head started to appear and disappear. That was very moving! She became harsh and ordered me to hold my breath while pushing instead of sighing heavily, in order to save energy. She apologized about that harshness afterwards, but I thought it was appropriate, for I needed a firm hand to stop me from drifting off the track. I usually like better to be able to go wild when in pain, but I thought it was O.K. to be a good girl and follow a line of action for the baby's sake.

My husband was supposed to receive the baby, but he didn't have time to get into the tank and my midwife did it instead, as the head was only half presenting when the whole body slipped out with a little hand by the face! They saw her looking around peacefully and curiously with wide open eyes at her new underwater realm. I was very surprised and de-lighted. She looked wholesome, all limbs, toes, and fingers! She was pink right away and practically without vernix and mucus in her nose and eyes, and well-ironed (without wrinkles). We emersed her head right away, as we wanted to bond, and she began to cry against my chest—but nothing serious. I whispered words of love and welcome to her. My hus-band was sharing my delight. It was such a touching moment! All pain had gone and this little angel had arrived instead, with the first singing birds of the dawn.

I was so surprised and elated that I cried out of joy and felt like a little child who is finally receiving the wonderful toy she had given up on. . . . In the rising dawn light, I felt I was witnessing my own rebirth. The whole day passed very slowly in that same enlightened atmosphere of love, love of the child, love of my husband, love of God, all connected and the same.

I feel that this experience, as trying as it was, was necessary, dying and rebirthing, and that no pain now can frighten or upset me in com-parison.

One of my dear friends, Patti, who at the time of her delivery lived at the very top of the Mayacamas Mountains, was due to deliver her fourth baby. Her second baby came out in forty-eight minutes, so I made sure I was close by and ready to assist. As we listened to Tahitian music on the radio late into the night, Patti danced the hula while in labor. I ducked outside to look at the Milky Way and smell the pines in the fresh mountain air. A hoot owl started calling as if to say that things had changed with Patti. I returned to find Patti's belly looking considerably lower. I checked her dilation. She was completely dilated (10 centimeters). Well, it didn't seem to phase her a bit, as she got back up and started dancing. She had no urges to push. I kept listening to the baby's heartbeat. All was well. Finally, after a half-hour went by, I asked her, "Well, are you ready to push yet?" She said she didn't feel a thing except contractions. So she decided to push anyway and out popped her baby, her fourth boy, Duane. This, I admit, is unusual, but it is an example as to the extremes to which the pushing urges of different women in different labors can go. On the other hand, when I was in labor, as hard as I tried, I couldn't stop myself from pushing.

In the winter of 1990 I was invited to Berlin, Germany, to teach the *hebamme* (midwives) to do water births. Several "ladies in waiting" were ready to meet with me and have their water births at the birth clinic of Maureen Amonis.

The first mother to go into labor was six feet tall with raven black hair. Her husband supported her in the bath, sometimes acting as a cushion, other times supporting her as she squatted. As she laid back against him during contractions, she remarked how much easier it was to relax in the water, rather than being on the hard bed that wouldn't mold to her shape. I noticed the difference. Her face looked softer, her body less tight. She didn't cry out as she did when she was in a less buoyant medium. She felt at ease at the clinic as she walked down the familiar halls that she had visited each month while her baby was growing in utero. Her midwife spoke softly and gently to her in German, words I couldn't understand but knew through the universal feelings and language of childbirth. Then, the baby's heartbeat went down too low to have a water birth safely. She needed to get out of the water. The mother simply stood up above the water and gave birth to a huge baby with the cord wrapped around the neck. We quickly unwrapped the cord and gave the baby a breath of oxygen. Both mother and baby were absolutely fine.

Although the couple wanted to have a water birth, they were not disappointed. They felt in control of their birth at the birth center and were delighted to have used the water for labor, let alone having the opportunity to have attempted a water birth.

Another German mother, who happened to be an obstetrician, decided she liked the familiarity and the comfort of her own home. While in labor she decided that she didn't want to give birth at the center. She wanted the privacy of her own home in case someone else might be laboring at the same time as she. So she phoned her midwife to come to her home instead of meeting her at the birthing center.

Most European bath tubs are longer, deeper, and wider than the modern American baths, so she was lucky and gave birth in her own bath. Her midwife came with all the equipment necessary for a home-birth and assisted her in the delivery of a lovely baby boy in her own home, in the water. The labor and delivery went very smoothly. Everyone was happy with the outcome, especially the midwife who was glad to have the experience of attending a water birth outside of the clinic setting.

A HOSPITAL WATER BIRTH

In Maidstone Hospital in Kent, England, midwives Linda Ford and Dianne Garland describe a hospital's first underwater delivery:

> Dawn lay back, relaxing so that her body floated in the water, until the next contraction when she commenced active pushing. She made excellent progress, the baby's head advancing steadily with each effort. I was astonished at the clarity of the water. The lights were dimmed yet we could still see the head quite clearly. As it crowned, I placed my hand upon it quite lightly and the head delivered. There was no cord around the neck. Dawn could see the baby's head and we all watched as rotation took place. I put my hands on the head and waited for a contraction. We all gazed at this most amazing sight. Just as we had been told, the baby made no attempt to open its eyes or to breathe. I was reminded of the pictures of the fetus in utero. With the next contraction the baby was delivered and as requested I gently guided her on to Dawn's breast. Only the baby's head was out of the water. She commenced breathing immediately; no suction was needed. She opened her eyes—she did not cry. I was astonished to see that even the hands and feet were pink (1989, p. 40).

In the same article, Dawn wrote of her own experience of giving birth in the hospital while in water:

> What bliss! My pain completely disappeared. I fancied I was on a Caribbean island, floating in a warm lagoon with the sun high in the sky and not a care in the world! My sense of control returned and I was able to deal with each contraction as it came. After a time I felt divorced from my surroundings, although still conscious of the other talking. I dozed between contractions. The next thing I remember is Linda telling me to open my eyes and look. There was my baby's head which had been delivered without me being aware of it. At that moment, seeing her peaceful, sleeping face, I was stunned to realise that I had been so relaxed and happy, I almost missed seeing the birth of my child. Incredible to think

that without any pain relief at all, the experience could be so pleasurable (1989, p. 40).

Not all births have the outcomes that women want. Amy Teresa and Tom were preparing to have a water birth, but the baby turned out to be breech. Here is Amy Teresa's story of her beautiful hospital birth.

The Birth of Gwendolyn Rose

We had both wanted our baby to be born at home with the support and guidance of our beloved midwife. However, it did not work out that way. It was Tuesday, around the 38th week, and our baby had not turned. Our midwife recommended that we get an ultrasound to make sure that everything was O.K. and possibly to find out why the baby was not turning.

On Wednesday the young doctor who did the ultrasound discovered that the baby was in fact breech, and she was so concerned (needlessly, fortunately) about her small size that she referred us to the high-risk pregnancy doctors.

On Friday we saw the high-risk doctor who found nothing wrong with the baby except that he thought it was the 34th week because of his standards of "normal." We knew he was wrong because we knew exactly when conception had happened. He also said that he never delivered breech babies naturally, so if the baby did not turn, we would have to have a C-section. We were not pleased about this possibility, but prepared ourselves for it emotionally and recognized that at least everyone would be healthy and safe.

On early Sunday morning at about 2 A.M. the waters broke. We called our midwife and doctor and quickly headed for the hospital. We had not as yet seriously considered the possibility of a hospital birth and thought that we had a couple of weeks more. So we ended up at the hospital in Berkeley with no hospital strategy.

We arrived at the hospital at around 3 A.M. with our 20-year-old son (who wanted to be with us during the birth) and two good friends. We were greeted by warm and friendly nurses. Our midwife met us there a short while later and was able to help us understand what was going on. I was hooked up to the fetal heart monitor which reassured me the baby was O.K. We saw the doctor on duty and, since the contractions were light and irregular and the baby was fine, we decided to wait and do nothing.

A few hours later another doctor came on duty and gave us a list of our choices. To our delight and surprise one of the choices was to have a vaginal delivery. He said that C-sections were boring and, since the baby was small, there shouldn't be any problem. He said he could try to turn her, but this option did not feel right to us, and we chose not to. Later we found out why. She had the umbilical cord wrapped twice around her neck and once around her arm, so turning her probably wouldn't have been successful and may have precipitated a crisis that would have resulted in a C-section. He also offered to give me a drug that would have delayed labor for twenty-four hours, thinking that she was slightly premature and the delay would give her lungs a chance to develop. However, he would be off duty by then, and the new doctor would not consider a vaginal delivery. Since we knew she was just small and not premature and since we wanted a vaginal delivery, we again decided to do nothing. We were always presented with all of the choices available to us and were allowed to choose what felt right to us without any pressure. Our midwife was there with us, and this was always a comfort and strength I would not have wanted to be without.

The birth itself was uncomplicated and miraculous. Our precious, perfect baby, Gwendolyn Rose, came into the world feet first with no drugs, surgery, or forceps, but with lots of ecstasy, love, and joy. Although somewhat disoriented, she did not even cry. Our midwife said it was a very low-stress birth for Gwen. The nurse who checked her said she was full term. She weighed in at just barely "normal"—5 pounds 1 ounce.

The only problem we had with the doctors was with the pediatrician who could not understand why we did not want a needle stuck into our baby. Finally, after a certain amount of tension and some very definite stubbornness on our part, he agreed to give the vitamin K to her orally.

Overall, we asked for what we wanted and were given it by a staff of exceptionally understanding doctors and nurses. Gwendolyn's birth showed us that the quality of experience which is possible with a home birth is also possible (although sometimes it may be necessary to be stubborn) when a hospital birth is necessary.

Roxanne wanted a water birth with her first child because she feared the pain of childbirth. She and her husband went to childbirth classes that did not depict labor and delivery in a realistic manner. Instead they were told that if the mother thinks of the pain in a positive light, the discomfort can be transcended. I believe this is possible and I have seen it happen, but if the mother is not prepared for all possibilities she may be setting herself up for circumstances that she never expected.

When Roxanne got into the water, she was only 4 centimeters dilated. Before getting into the tank, she was yelling, screaming, and carrying on. I had never seen a woman laboring in a home setting so close to hysteria. None of the support and advice that we gave her was working. When she got into the water, she did calm down; it soothed her and she became more relaxed. This brought on stronger and more frequent contractions.

"I'm not supposed to be feeling this," she moaned.

She fought the sensations and continued bellowing. My assistant and I tried to teach her to breathe and surrender to the pain; to look at labor as good, helping her baby to come out.

"This wasn't supposed to hurt," she would scream.

At long last she wore herself out and became so tired that she couldn't fight any more. Roxanne finally let her body work as it needed to, realizing that there was going to be a certain amount of discomfort. After that she became calmer, enjoying the water and her freedom of movement. When she would leave the tank, she would tighten up again and would start carrying on. After twenty-four hours, she gave birth to Mary. The pushing stage lasted only an hour. The 10-pound girl was born with clenched fists and a grimaced face. This is *very* atypical of a water baby. Most are born so relaxed they appear to be asleep. My first inclination was to bring her up out of the water, but her parents objected, thinking that the water would calm her. In most cases one or two minutes would enable the baby to relax and adjust to her new environment. We brought her out of the water after one minute. She was still tight, unable to relax. Putting her to the breast didn't help either. Mary was returned to the water with only her face left above the surface. Mom swayed her gently back and forth and sang the songs that Mary heard in the womb. This helped, and she slowly unfolded her tightly clenched body. It was the first time baby Mary relaxed and the first time Roxanne really relaxed.

While examining Roxanne's vagina, after the birthing process was complete, I found a tear in her perineum and stitched her up.

A few days later Roxanne and her husband informed me how angry they were that Roxanne had torn her perineum. This was one of the main reasons why they had wanted a water birth. I, on the other hand, couldn't believe how naive this couple was in believing they could control an act of nature.

Eventually, the parents realized what a beautiful birthing experience they had had and telephoned to tell me so. A first-time mom who gives birth to a 10-pound baby usually has a harder time, especially if dogmatic expectations are prevalent during the labor. It is best to let nature take its course and to set aside any preconceived ideas on what labor should or shouldn't be like.

FATHERS' STORIES

Here some fathers who have actively participated in the labor and delivery of their children discuss how the event represented one of the most fulfilling times in their lives. This first story by Jeff René depicts not only how the father participated in the labor and delivery of his water babies, but also how he built their tanks, which led him to build tanks for others who wanted water births.

In 1984, we decided to explore the possibility of water birth for our expected child. I had become aware of Igor Charkowsky's work in 1969 and had followed the scant reporting on water birth in the press and journals from that time. With this general awareness in hand, we needed to decide on two important elements of the birth; a midwife/educator, to complete our education on methods and potentials of water birth, and to be our monitor and advisor at the birth; and "the equipment," what we needed to buy, rent, or construct to create a quality water birth environment in our home. The first element was easy; we found our midwife through a homebirth network. In her we found a skilled midwife, willing to allow us as much control in our birth as we were willing to accept, a good teacher, a light spirit at our birth, and a good friend. Each couple or single mother comes to the selection of a midwife with different needs and expectations. It's an important decision, to find the balance in personality, skills, and trust that meets your needs! Start early! Take your time! The second element, the equipment, was more difficult. In the end we built our own tub system to meet our needs.

In our birth experience, letting things progress of their own accord seemed the safest course to follow. There are perspectives on birth methods that advocate removing the baby from both the mother's birth canal and the water as quickly as possible as the safer way to proceed. These attitudes are rooted in a lack of information and experience; they may create dangers.

During the birth of my first child born in the water, Colette, a 9½-pound baby, it was necessary to unwrap the umbilical cord from her neck while in the water. Her face seemed pensive, her eyes and mouth open. We waited perhaps forty seconds for the next contraction; then her shoulders cleared, her arms cleared, and with only gentle assistance, she was out to her waist. We could easily have pulled her clear from mom at that point, but we saw no need. She spread her arms out from her sides, first to the 180 degree point, then a little farther; mouth and eyes still open, the tension and pensive look on her face disappeared. She reached one hand up out of the water and was tracking the sounds of people moving around the tub. Another forty seconds and with the next contraction she was clear of mom. A solid trickle of blood followed her into the water. We brought Colette up when the blood in the water began interfering with our monitoring of her facial features.

Our second child born in the water, Maia, was an entirely different experience. At about 5 centimeters dilation, with contractions just under five minutes apart, mom experienced a tremendous change in chemical or hormonal balance. She vomited and evacuated in a moment, and said she wanted to give a push. One push and Maia was born, sound asleep, curled on the bottom of the tub. Her mouth open, she tried to remain asleep for perhaps thirty seconds before she had opened her eyes wide, looking over her new environment. Perhaps forty-five seconds had passed from birth to the use of her arms, then one leg, then both. We brought Maia out of the water within two minutes.

These two stories are meant to describe the fact that each birth will unfold, for each mother, and each new baby in its own timing and way. For the parents and medical backup to establish standards for the environment and situations that might arise in the birth as their guide, and to then observe and monitor carefully, seems the safest and best method.

I think the time of physical opening in the water is very important to the child. This first unrestrained physical experience outside of the mother is a reference point for physical development. It establishes a wider paradigm for physicality in an environment that is familiar and supportive. It is in the same manner as visual bonding with the parents, a touchstone throughout the life of a person. To enter into the work of preparation and training towards the birth of a child, and to leave out consideration for the child's physical opening in the world seems an unnecessary restriction and loss. I don't in any way advocate time trials, seeing how long you can go—certainly, even with good strong umbilical pulse, there is over time, a diminishing supply of oxygen. It is a matter of observing the situation and if there is no reason to interrupt this physical opening, then let it be.

During our first water birth, after Colette was clear, mom didn't have another contraction for perhaps twenty-five minutes. This led to a wonderful bonding time for baby and father. I have suggested this to couples for years, that during the magic half hour of visual bonding at birth, that dad be primary, not to exclude mom, but to make use of an excellent opportunity. Mothers have plenty of fine bonding time during the first weeks and through nursing, but in many cases fathers do not. In our case, this time allowed a relationship to develop such that either parent could soothe and comfort—and enhanced the peace of our family.

These ideas on the birth environment are about this point—there is a psychological environment at the birth that we bring to the birth. It is healthy to begin the process of our training by allaying nagging fears: can my baby drown, is there more chance of infection, etc.? Research and educate yourselves. Establish the limits of your birth method within which you are comfortable—you can't take anyone else's word on this. It always scares me when people tell me they never worried about any part of water birth, or that they would rather not hear of any dangerous potential. By educating and then working within ourselves, we can bring ease to our children's birth.

This process of working toward the birth of our children provides a wonderful window on our own lives and births. If we pay attention, it is interesting, the kind of things that emerge.

This journey started out for me as a kind of affinity, the letting out of a long breath on seeing a film of Charkowsky's work in the late sixties. Through two joyous and empowering births, that corroborated my initial response, to an adventure in equipment building and sharing resources.

The people who came to my door for water birth tanks through the years cut across all the political, racial, and social lines. They were doctors, lawyers, policemen, a submarine commander, hippies, artists, small-business people, single moms, etc., and they generally shared one hope: that they could provide the best and safest situation in their home, to facilitate the least traumatic birth possible for their children. If any group predominated, it was the medical professionals who had made the decision to birth at home. They weren't on the whole people who had bought into any particular philosophy about birth; they had reasonable questions and fears and were willing to work out the problems. They wanted to have control over decision making at their children's births and were willing to assume the responsibility for those choices. They gave me a sense that we are all unified in our basic human concerns, and that it is our humanness that we have to allow to reemerge.

Finally, the way of the birth permeates the life; our choices have impact beyond our understanding; trust your own feelings about the birth of your children, educate yourself, and work carefully.

Jeffrey Lee René

Another father writes of his participation and bonding with their new son.

When my wife, Gina, approached me about having a homebirth, I was against it because we had medical insurance that wouldn't cover a non-AMA delivery. I also felt that the hospital nearest us was "in with the times" because of its home-style birthing rooms. This was not going to be one of those on your back, feet in the stirrups, slap the butt, and tell the husband it's a boy types of births. Why spend an extra $900 for a midwife when the hospital, which has a wonderful birthing program, was already paid for?

If we had no insurance, a homebirth would have been the way to go. Not only because it would be far less expensive than a hospital birth, but for all the other reasons, too. As I was making my stand, Gina brought up the underwater birth idea. This meant that we would have to shell out another $250 to rent a birthing tank. I was thinking to myself: what's next, rented lighting and sitar players?

I strongly believed that the pregnancy was of the utmost importance and *where* the baby was actually delivered was relatively insignificant. I watch television. I've seen the Indian woman squatting next to the tree stump, the city mother on the side of the freeway and the 911 birth over the phone. These babies came out great. As I added this up, $900 plus $250 plus a guesstimated $350 for miscellaneous incidentals, that was $1,500 that we could have saved if we took the show to the hospital.

After around month four of our pregnancy and after really listening to Gina, I finally surrendered and gave my consent. You see, although this was my first pregnancy, it was Gina's third. Our other two children, Nathan and Rochelle, who are 12 and 10 years old, were born the caesarean way.

Gina felt that she was naive in her youth and therefore manipulated into the drugging, surgery, and intense recuperation that becomes part of the caesarean package. This time, eleven years later, well-read and more astute, she wanted to birth our baby on her own terms, at home, where she could have complete control, and vaginally, like it's supposed to be. She also felt that a water birth would greatly enhance the home-birth and ensure a smooth delivery.

During our pregnancy, Gina studied hard and I browsed (relatively speaking) through information regarding home and water birth. We did not do this haphazardly. We turned the light on these methods and sincerely prepared ourselves. We topped off our education with a beautiful drive to Glen Ellen where Susanna gave us a private seminar on water births. This preparation eliminated fears, and through our newfound knowledge we became ready to respond and strong enough to go through with this venture.

Renting a birthing tank was rather easy (especially for me since Gina did all the leg work). She found it through "Waterbirth International" out of Oregon. For a $250 rental fee, they sent us an inflatable rubber water tank, electric air pump, heater, water siphon, and a water thermometer. Our rental agreement allowed us to keep the tank for one month. We set up the tank in a back room which became our birthing room.

On October 4, 1992, the big event arose with the dawn—it was labor day. Gina began using the water tank at around 10 A.M. The warm salted water and buoyancy helped to relieve her labor pains and set her at ease. The more intense the labor got, the more she used the tank.

Our midwives had never been at a water birth. Although they went along with this and understood the benefits of warm water during labor, I could tell that they were a bit concerned about the *under*water birth.

As of 8 P.M. on "labor day," Gina was spending most of her time in the birthing tank. Around 9 P.M., Gina got out of the tank for a vaginal exam and it happened—her water broke.

Now it was my turn to get my feet wet. I stripped down naked and in all my modesty got into the tank with my wife. As Gina was pushing and paining, I was giving the play-by-play on our baby's progress to the birthing team.

Gina, who was attempting a VBAC eleven years after the fact, was doing great. Our other two children, the two midwives, Melinda (Gina's sister), and I were all doing what we could to facilitate this miracle.

I reported that the baby's head was up against the vaginal exit. Gina pushed and her vagina bulged. She pushed again and the head came half way out. All the while, what I could feel with my hands became everyone else's eyes as the darkened room and murky water clouded our vision. One more push and our baby's head was out.

With the midwife supporting Gina's back, Rochelle harboring blankets against her warm tummy, Nathan's watchful eye on the clock we had pre-set to the exact time, Melinda on the camera with high-speed film, the other midwife's hands in the water blindly cupping our baby's head (along with my hands), a full minute went by and the rest of the baby's body was still not out.

As far as the midwife was concerned, one minute with the baby's head under water was long enough. She wanted to see with her eyes what was going on. She ordered Gina out of the tank: "Let's get her out of the tank!"

At that moment our baby shot out like a torpedo. I caught the child and immediately brought it to the surface. This was a pre-planned maneuver. Since none of us had ever witnessed a water birth, we didn't want to risk the baby gulping any water.

As soon as I brought the baby to the surface, it cried its first breath. I remember sitting next to my panting wife; we were wet, warm, and secure. Our baby was crying and in its mother's arms. The situation was timeless.

After a couple of minutes had passed, Gina looked and saw that she had delivered a boy. It wasn't long before our son began to nurse. We sat there in the warm water and dimly lit room and cuddled with our newborn as he ate and ate.

Every now and then the midwife had me check the pulsing umbilical cord. We didn't want to cut it until after it had stopped pulsating. As the moments passed, our baby, cradled in his mother's arms, sucked milk like there was no tomorrow. The midwife asked me to check the cord again. It was still pulsing. She expressed her surprise, stating that she had never seen a cord pulsate for forty-five minutes. This shocked me because it seemed like it had only been ten minutes since our son was born. At Kimberly's suggestion, I cut the cord even though it was still throbbing. We then took our baby out of the water and began with the post-birth exercises.

Our healthy son, Dominic Leigh Tassinari, weighed in at 9 pounds 4 ounces, and was 21 inches long. Gina and I are convinced that the wetness, buoyancy, splashing sounds, and the warmth of the water birth greatly eased the delivery of our large VBAC boy. The water birth seemed so natural. A bed birth now seems dry and resistive.

Since Dominic's birth, I take him in the shower with me every morning. I hold him in my arms as the warm water sprinkles our bodies for ten to twenty minutes. I sing him songs and he falls asleep.

A TWIN WATER BIRTH

The birth story of twins Kavi and Teja is a remarkable story as seen through the eyes of a mother/midwife. Attempting twins at home is controversial, and adding water as the medium of birth may raise more than a few eyebrows. This story is told by a woman who knew what she wanted for her birth. As a professional, she was aware of the taboos of twins at home. She also knew in what parameters to work; what things were safe and when, if necessary, to go to the hospital. Her story is full of strength and empowerment, dispelling many of the fears surrounding giving birth to twins.

I had known for years that I wanted to birth in the water. As a midwife, I had witnessed the water helping women relax and be more comfortable. For myself, I remembered that when my first three labors began, I immediately got into the bathtub and did not want to get out, so I knew that water was my ally for birth. In May, near the beginning of the third trimester, I finished with the births I was to attend before my birthing. I had planned to take those last months and focus on my own pregnancy. With a due date of August 13, it meant being able to stay home during the summer heat. I was so glad that I had made this plan from the beginning because events were about to show me how necessary it would be to nurture my pregnancy.

I participated in my prenatal care, but had regular check-ins with the midwives with whom I work. At 27 weeks, I had a growth spurt of 8 centimeters in one week (1 centimeter of growth per week is average.) [*Author's note:* Peggy is speaking of the measurement of her fundal growth per week.] There was so much amniotic fluid it was impossible to palpate well at all. [*Author's note:* Palpate means to feel the mother's belly in order to feel how the baby is lying.] I waited a week until our next midwifery meeting. I had a strong sense of well-being and waited for the truth to reveal itself in its own right time. Then the day I turned 28 weeks, when the uterus is more clearly available for palpation, and which happened to be the full moon in Gemini, there they were—two babies—one head down in my pelvis and one seemingly smaller breech, with his head under my heart, a good birthing position. Two midwives listening with two fetoscopes simultaneously confirmed what hands had felt—two beings with two very distinct heartbeats growing within.

I was strongly supported in my birth plans by my husband, Will, and our midwives, who saw twins as quite acceptable for homebirth. We worked together as guardians to this normal experience. With twins it is optimal that the first baby be head down, and larger. A smaller, second baby being breech is not a huge concern because the birth canal is opened by the first baby, providing plenty of room for the next baby who is often born quickly.

The babies' positions were palpated often and never moved out of optimal birthing position, an affirmation to us all. I was also glad to hear that my hematocrit at 32 weeks was 43.0! [*Author's note:* The hematocrit is the volume of erythrocytes in a given blood volume. A safe hematocrit for a home birth is 36.0. Lower than that may mean anemia.] This was a good sign that I could carry them in a healthy way until they were full term, as anemia can cause premature birth. My goal was to intelligently evaluate all the information I had, clinical and intuitive, and everything pointed to a safe homebirth. I was not drawn in any way to consider other birth plans, and was convinced that these babies wanted to be born in the sanctity of our home, in the water.

With increased growth, my pregnancy became more physically taxing, but never debilitating. I surrendered my activity level, staying home more and giving up even routine household tasks. The love and support of my family and friends helped make this possible and relatively smooth. I was never on bed rest, but naturally found I needed to lie down more and more for energy and comfort's sake. The truth was that during the last month, I couldn't drive because I did not fit behind the wheel of my car with the seat all the way back. Also the last time I drove, I experienced strong Braxton-Hicks contractions that distracted me. Although I did not fear I would have a premature birth, I knew I needed to be wise to help these babies mature to full term. It was time to be home. I measured 54 centimeters at 38 weeks. (Forty cm is normal for a single pregnancy at full term of 40 weeks.)

My labor started August 1 at 5:00 A.M. I was delighted. My goal, set the day after I found out about the twins, was to get my pregnancy into August when they would be 38 weeks. I had actually predicted the birth being August 1 two months earlier. I awakened Will to help me go to the bathroom (that process sometimes needed help by then), and I felt a pop and slowly leaking waters. Two of my three previous labors had started this way with contractions beginning within minutes. Will went to get the midwife who was staying on the land. She took heart tones of both babies which were good, and the three of us walked to the house. I knew I was in labor—there was so much energy my teeth were chattering and I was shaky all over. The midwife got the tub ready as I wanted to get in the water as soon as possible. Contractions were getting strong.

I was so glad to get into the water. I immediately felt more relaxed and able to move. I was huge with these babies and found moving awkward in full gravity. For me, the water was an incredible gift. The other midwives arrived. Our daughters were awakened. The room was filled with love—love for one another, love for these two beings who came to be with us. This love truly sustained me as labor proceeded.

At 8 centimeters dilation, the contractions got farther apart. New positions in the water applied the head to the cervix better, but did not increase dilation. I had been feeling short of breath. My lungs were fairly compressed and I longed for fresh air. With much help I walked outside into the yard. It still seemed that I could not get enough air, but I loved being outside and standing up. Walking and rocking my pelvis aided dilation. It was hard to walk up the stairs to the house, but once I was in the water, I felt better again, like transformation. The anterior lip of the cervix melted away in a few contractions and I was ready to push.

This labor was quite different from my others; two babies and the over-distension of my uterus made for less effective contractions than I had ever had before. My other labors had always had steady progress, and pushing contractions were efficient and effective. Now, as I was ready to push, the time I had been awaiting, my pushing contractions did not seem strong, and pushing on two babies felt awkward, like I was pushing on the top baby to push out the bottom one. I needed gravity and found that getting on my knees, leaning on the tub and on Will, then pushing worked best. Each contraction was an act of will, not an uncontrollable urge. My uterus felt like it was working at about 50 percent, although that is just my perception. The water definitely helped me be in the optimal birthing position. I was so heavy, I am sure I could not have maintained it without the buoyancy. I affirmed "I can" as each contraction began and put all my strength into each push.

It was a very conscious labor for me as my contractions were not sweeping me away for the birth. I worked hard pushing and put my finger in my vagina between pushes to feel how far the head had come down. Then I realized that the head had moved behind my pubic bone and I resolved to move it past the bone with the next contraction. I called on the Angels of Birth and drew on the strength of the ritual of my Blessing Way. I remembered all the mothers who have given birth and found the power coming through me that could do this work. With that contraction the head came from behind the pubic bone and was birthed. I marveled at the thought of my baby being partly born and partly still inside me, yet still in the water, his familiar environment. It seemed so natural and optimal for him.

Three minutes later the next contraction brought the shoulders and Kavi was born, an 8-pound baby! He was born at 10:23 A.M., five hours and twenty-three minutes after labor began. The midwife caught him and brought him out of the water immediately. We had agreed to this ahead of time because I wanted to hold him and give him the full grace of gradually experiencing breathing while still receiving oxygen from his cord. He was left with his umbilical cord pulsing for only one minute and then it was clamped and cut in case his twin sibling shared some circulation, and he was not allowed to nurse in case it would cause inappropriate contractions for his twin. Kavi came out of the water and breathed within moments—they seemed so short—and then our oldest daughter, Melissa, rocked him by the woodstove as we prepared for the next birth.

It was a lot of surrender for me to let go of Kavi so soon, but I was amazed how fast I turned my attention to the birth of the next baby. Our midwife was his guardian, carefully monitoring his heart tones, and after Kavi was born, she used her hands on my belly to guide him straight down into the pelvis to prevent a transverse lie. I felt that he and I were very safe in her caring, competent hands.

The midwife did an internal exam—an extremely uncomfortable experience, even as gentle as the midwife was, because of the stretching and bruising of the tissues of the cervix and birth canal from the first birth. I remember saying, "I can't believe I have to do this again." But I also had much conscious determination to birth the second baby as soon as possible. The midwife's exam discovered a bulging water bag around a head! We had been prepared for a breech. I thought it was fine either way.

My labor had essentially stopped. I was only having slight twinges for contractions and pushing with them did nothing. The head was high and my tired uterus was not bringing it down. I tried homeopathy, sitting up for gravity, and even allowing Kavi to nurse a bit. I felt totally normal like I wasn't in labor, and only slight contractions resumed.

We all wanted the second baby born and I really wanted the membranes ruptured. I thought I would be most comfortable for this procedure on a nearby futon. I was wrong. I forgot about gravity after being weightless in the tub. Lying down was excruciating for my back and ligaments. This made me realize how fortunate I'd been to birth in the water. I finally got onto my knees, leaned on the window seat, and the membranes were ruptured. I immediately went from no contractions or birthing energy to pushing as the baby's head came down onto the cervix.

I thought the baby was coming out. The tub was only a few steps away, but getting there seemed impossible. I didn't want to move. I feared getting into an awkward position half way there with the baby coming out. This fear was more based on my precipitous birth of Padma five and a half years before than on present circumstances. I birthed Padma in less than two hours without pushing at all, an extremely intense experience.

Our midwife and homeopath said to me, "Where do you want to birth?" I replied that I didn't think I could get over to the tub. Then she said, "Peggy, where does your baby want to be born?" I immediately said, "In the water." Will, who shared my strong belief that our babies wanted to be born through water, helped me get into the tub before the next contraction. Once there I felt light again and as comfortable as one gets under the circumstances. What a blessing.

Once again my contractions were only semi-effective, but pushing a smaller baby through an already expanded birth canal was easier. Again I pushed out the head and then was between contractions. Another baby was in those timeless moments between two worlds and embraced by water. After three minutes, I had another contraction and pushed with all of my strength, but he was not moving. He needed the midwife to help birth an arm before his body could be born. I was elated when Teja finally birthed five minutes after I reentered the tub. I could see he was another good-sized baby, seven pounds, birthed at 11:28, one hour and five minutes after his brother. Fifteen pounds of baby in all! He was also brought out of the water right away in deference to his brother, so I could finish the birth and be with both of them as soon as possible. Teja was given to our 12-year-old daughter, Rohanna, to join his brother by the woodstove during the birth of the placenta.

I got out of the tub to walk the few steps to the futon to birth the placenta and hemorrhaged half way there. Our midwife skillfully and gently held my uterus and I stabilized. I experienced a partial separation of the placenta that proved difficult to deal with for a while. We tried herbs, homeopathy, and nursing. I bled again and was getting shocky. Still the placenta did not birth. Something needed to happen soon.

I strongly felt that there was an Energy that would help me birth the placenta, but I did not know how to access it. At first I kept trying to find it within myself, but it seemed elusive. Then in my shocky state, I was actually visualizing it as being in the cupboard where I kept my homeopathics. We were certain that a large part of the placenta was still attached to the uterine wall. Finally, as hope of birthing the placenta without medical help was diminishing, the midwife gave me a new remedy, and the placenta was released and fell out into my hand. It was amazing how the remedy changed the energy. I went from being shocky and stuck to delivering the placenta and my mind cleared immediately. I am so grateful.

I write this nearly three months after the birth. The postpartum time has been blissful, exhausting, and very blessed. Twins are literally two handfuls, and to care for them requires group effort. A family with twins needs a lot of support, and we have been blessed with meals, love, and helping hands. The first two nights I don't remember sleeping at all, as Will and I handed babies back and forth to change, nurse, and rock. Days and nights seemed only slightly better than this for two and a half months. Just now is life looking realistic again.

I am grateful that they are healthy, vibrant babies and I have been able to nurse them totally. I have to be conscious of supporting my milk supply with food and fluids as I am not particularly well rested. It seems like I nurse the babies all the time, sometimes individually, sometimes at the same time. I want them to have the quality of care I gave my singleton children, and I forgive myself daily for those times I must put one baby down to care for the other and for those things I cannot do for other family members because of the twins. But, all in all, Kavi and Teja are getting their needs met in a loving way. Our children and friends help tremendously, and it has served to make our family and extended family ever closer.

I am grateful for this beautiful birth experience. I give thanks that Teja and Kavi were able to make the sacred transition from womb to earth in an environment filled with love and with an absence of fear. I am grateful to my sister midwives who facilitated the sacrament of birth for us in a holy and loving way. I write this in hope that by sharing this experience it will contribute toward demystifying twin births so that it will not be routinely considered "high risk" and in need of medical intervention, but instead will be seen as a normal, healthy condition that can be greatly enhanced by birthing in water at home.

APPENDIX A:
1982 FINAL REPORT TO THE
PEOPLE OF CALIFORNIA

During my research, I obtained this study directed by California as-semblyperson John Vasconcellos. The report was a result of two years of research by a California select commission investigating the causes and prevention of violence. I have included this part of the study be-cause of the increasing amount of seemingly recreational violence that is rapidly becoming part of our culture. This study is one of the few that I have come upon that says "yes," the way in which we enter the world can make a difference!

OUNCES OF PREVENTION—TOWARD UNDERSTANDING OF THE CAUSES OF VIOLENCE
State of California Commission on Crime Control and Violence Prevention

THE BIRTH EXPERIENCE PARENT/INFANT BONDING

A. The Birth Experience

Findings:

1. It will probably remain impossible—given the limits of predictive science and the vast array of conditions occurring after birth which influence a person's personality and behavior—to trace developmental problems and violent tendencies in later life directly to a person's birth experience. It is possible, however, to identify conditions surrounding birth which may contribute subsequently to parenting disorders (child

abuse or neglect) and/or developmental problems on the part of the child.

2. Although no direct link is known to exist between the birth experience and violent behavior, the events surrounding birth influence subsequent relations between parent(s) and child, and thus affect the child's emotional, cognitive and behavioral development. Accordingly, the Commission believes that a positive birth experience—one that is gentle, loving, and non-traumantic—increases the likelihood of healthy child development.

B. Early Parent–Infant Bonding

Findings:

1. A human being develops a number of affectional bonds throughout his or her lifetime. As unique attachments between two people that are specific and endure over time, these relationships bind together various individuals in a society, and greatly influence a person's sense of self and ability to respond appropriately to others. The maternal–infant attachment is but one of these relationships. However, the fact that it is crucial to the infant's survival and development suggests it may be the strongest of human bonds. Ideally, the bonding process between mothering person(s) and child commences at birth and evolves over time into an ever deeper emotional attachment (Klaus and Kennell, 1976; Harlow and Means, 1978).

a. Most research on early bonding addresses the mother–infant relationship. However, fathers allowed early, extended contact report stronger feelings of affection and "connectedness" with their newborns and evidence greater participation in their child's caretaking and nurturing than do limited-contact fathers (Greenberg and Morris, 1974).

2. Early parent–infant bonding is facilitated by a healthy birth.

An optimally healthy birth experience:

a. is family-centered, loving, natural, gentle, and non-traumatic;

b. actively involves parents in their child's birth, in its planning and facilitation; and

c. includes the presence of a supportive person for the woman in labor—be it father, friend, or trained assistant.

[There are, of course, situations wherein an optimally healthy birth is impossible for medical reasons. Furthermore, parental preference may exclude certain birth practices. Decisions regarding alternative birth procedures, therefore, should be made by the physician and potential parents on a case-by-case basis.]

3. Newborns are extremely alert and receptive to stimulation immediately following birth. Thus, from birth there exists an important opportunity for reciprocal interaction between infant and parent(s). It

is during the hours and days following delivery that the affectional bond between parent(s) and child initially asserts itself (Brazelton, 1978; Klaus and Kennell, 1976).

[This is not meant to imply that parent(s) and child who are separated after birth lose the opportunity to bond. In most instances, bonding is merely delayed temporarily.]

4. A mother who is heavily sedated or unconscious is unable to initiate interaction with her baby or respond to her baby's advances. Sedatives and anesthetics given to the mother during birth may collect in the baby's bloodstream and central nervous system causing less responsive or depressed infant behavior (Brazelton, 1965; Brazelton and Robey, 1970). Interaction between infant and parent(s) may thus be hindered and the early bonding process temporarily hindered.

5. Extended contact between parent(s) and infant in the hours, days and weeks immediately following birth, such as that afforded by hospital rooming-in facilities, home or neighborhood-facility birth, may promote the development of an affectional bond between them and thus enhance their subsequent relationship. Extended early contact, however, is not sufficient to prevent parenting disorders in most cases; and its absence is not usually associated with demonstrably harmful effects (O'Connor et al., 1980).

6. Although hospitals increasingly allow prolonged contact, many hospitals still routinely separate newborn and parents except for feedings.

7. Extreme isolation and prolonged separation from parents is routine for newborns treated in the Intensive Care Nursery.

　　a. Current state regulations increase the potential for over-use of intensive care nurseries because licensure depends on the number of patients treated. [*Author's note:* This could mean that the nurseries get more funding the more that they are used.]

Recommendations:

1. Educate prospective parents regarding the significance of the birth experience, and:

　　a. disseminate information to the public and to medical personnel about alternative birth practices which maximize parental involvement, family intimacy, and natural delivery;

　　b. promote education as to the importance of early affectional bonding between parents and their newborn child;

　　c. educate fathers as to the *responsibility* to fully participate in the family and in the birth, care, and nurturance of their children; and

　　d. educate fathers as to their right to full participation in the family and in the birth, care and nurturance of their children.

2. Encourage extended contact between parent(s) and the newborn immediately after birth.

3. Discourage unnecessary use of intensive care nursery facilities (which by definition separate parents and infant).

a. Encourage efforts to maximize parent–infant contact in intensive care nursery facilities.

4. Encourage parental leave from work for both mother and father following the birth of their child.

5. Encourage childbirth alternatives (in both birth procedures and facilities) which offer safe care in a loving, family environment where prospective parents (both mother and father) are active participants in planning for and carrying out delivery.

6. Undertake research to further assess the possibility of a connection between the birth experience and subsequent violent behavior.

C. Minimal Brain Damage

Findings:

1. There is evidence that minimal brain damage, perhaps sustained at birth, is associated with learning disabilities and attention deficit disorders which, in turn, may be associated with juvenile delinquency and adult criminality.

2. The brain of the fetus is rapidly developing during the period of time that surrounds birth and is thus extremely vulnerable to damage from drugs and surgical procedures administered to mother (Haire, 1980). Obstetric intervention procedures (including drugs and surgery) may increase the risk of neurological injury to the infant.

a. Sedatives (other than general anesthetics) given to the mother during labor are transferred to the fetus and result in a less responsive newborn. Findings remain inconclusive as to whether drug-related, decreased responsiveness causes permanent retardation or brain damage (Brazelton and Robey, 1970).

[*Author's note:* General anesthetics have the same result as sedatives.]

b. Surgical intervention procedures such as elective cesarean section, forceps removal and amniotomy pose a risk to the infant of neurological injury and minimal brain damage.

c. The apgar test (most commonly given newborns) to assess their neurological competence (according to heart rate, respiration, muscle tone and skin color) may be an inadequate means of measuring subtle or minimal brain damage (Coletti, 1979; Haire, 1980; Brazelton and Robey, 1970).

3. Poor nutrition or substance abuse by a mother during pregnancy can affect the fetus and result in low birth weight and premature birth, and abnormal or retarded brain development.

Recommendations:

1. Educate medical professionals and prospective parents that birth is a healthy process in which high technology, medical intervention procedures and intra-labor drugs need not be routinely administered.

2. Require, for the purpose of data collection and treatment, that a copy of the mother's complete obstetric record (labor record, nursing notes, medication record, X-rays, etc.) be made a permanent part of the child's medical record. (Sensitive, confidential, non-medical information should be excluded.)

3. Require attending health care professionals to inform a woman during her pregnancy of the drugs and procedures they plan to use during delivery and of the risks involved.

4. Undertake research to:

   a. assess the unintended, potentially adverse effects on newborns of high technology and intra-labor drugs; and

   b. develop neurological assessment tools to ascertain, more accurately than is currently possible, subtle, minimal brain damage and subsequent dysfunction.

D. At-Risk Parents and Children

Findings:

1. Parents at-risk for parenting problems (manifested by varying degrees of child abuse and neglect) often are *identifiable prior to and soon after the child's birth.* Many factors combine to indicate potential parenting problems. Among them are: mother's age, drug usage, and history of abusive behavior (Roth, 1980).

   a. Hospital staff, medical professionals, and community health care workers are in a position to identify at-risk parents before and after the child's birth.

2. Premature infants are at greater risk for abuse than full-term infants (Hunter et al., 1978).

   a. Intensive care nursery staff are in a position to effect early identification and intervention because the extended contact with parents provides the opportunity of observing parental interaction with the premature infant.

Recommendations:

1. Encourage the inclusion of prenatal health education and alternative birthing information in public school curricula, and recommend its inclusion for private schools.

2. Provide health care facilitators with training in early identification of and intervention with at-risk parents.

3. Support and expand existing early identification and intervention programs.

4. Provide prenatal support, educational, and diagnostic services to all prospective parents, particularly those known to fit at-risk criteria. These services should be readily available, offered in communities and neighborhoods, at minimal or no cost.

5. Provide parents identified by hospital personnel as being at-risk to abuse or neglect their child with follow-up attention and support services.

APPENDIX B:
THE BLESSING WAY

For most women in the United States, the baby shower is part of the pregnancy. The gathering of close friends and relatives to shower the mother with gifts and well wishes is, to some degree, a ritual. Another ritual which some pregnant women are reviving is a version of the Native American rite of passage, the Blessing Way, which Navajos use to mark their passage through different stages of life, such as puberty. Pregnant women use the Blessing Way to empower them in their last few months of pregnancy and enable them to give birth with the strength of a lioness.

Why is a ritual performed? Rituals bring the participants together as a group to express different levels of human consciousness. A ritual brings forth images and visions, evoking memories, feelings, fears, joys, and good intentions and wishes for the group or an individual. The ritual may also be considered a prayer. Through rituals we become healers and creators, and we get in touch with our consciousness and our wishes. Once this step is taken we may go on to the next one: to enjoy it, purge it, study it, or just do it.

A ritual helps to ease and define our transformations. Ritual, then, may be seen as a loud prayer, a support for the person who is going through transition. An ancient theory behind the use of ritual is that, while in ceremony, an individual or a collective passes from one state to another through a process of crisis or ordeal to a higher place.

The Blessing Way is usually attended by close friends and family. It has been traditional for only women friends to be present, but some women also ask their close male friends to participate. These men contribute much support for the pregnant woman. Close friends empower the pregnant woman, bestowing good-will and love upon her and her baby. This love helps her feel the power in sisterhood and, as the case may be, in brotherhood.

The midwife who is catching the baby customarily leads the ceremony. This ceremony helps establish and deepen the spiritual bond between the midwife and the pregnant mother, allowing the mother to find her feelings and to understand her midwife's feelings about the sanctity of birth. In one sense the ritual provides the groundwork for the coming labor. It can bring visions and enhance the mother's intuition, enabling her to trust that the intuitive wisdom will infuse her while laboring and giving birth.

To begin the ritual, some time should be taken to create a sacred space. The midwife can explain the space and the reason for the ritual to all the participants, welcome everyone and initiate singing or chanting. The ceremony may take an hour or two and should not be rushed. Being relaxed and calm will help the spirit to touch everyone, whatever that spirit may be for each individual. Ideally, the ritual should be performed in the pregnant mother's home a month to two weeks before the baby is due. This will help establish a feeling of sanctity and security in the environment where the mother is to give birth.

The participants may want to bring their talismans—that is, items that mean something special to them, items that represent strength, good-will, and courage. Everyone is asked to sit in a circle because the circle represents life's circle, our planet, and our family circle. In this circle, we are all equal; no one is in front, and no one is behind.

The next part of the Blessing Way ritual is to acknowledge the symbolism of the four directions. The midwife should explain the meaning of the four directions. It is preferable that the pregnant mother be previously counseled on the symbolism of the four directions and that she choose the four persons who are to represent each of the four directions. The four directions are North, South, East, and West. They can be found with a compass, with the persons chosen for the directions sitting in their represented spots.

The North. The element is the earth, and the season is winter. The North symbolizes old age and wisdom, and is represented by the crone or wise-woman. The color is green or black, and the time of day representing the northern direction is midnight. Some consider the North to be the most powerful direction. Along with this comes the power of silence, which is mysterious and unseen. The North gives the power to keep silent and to speak appropriately. The animal is the bull or buffalo, and the five-pointed star or the pentacle represents this direction of wisdom.

The South. The element is fire, and the season is the summer. Noon is the time of day representing this direction. Some believe that the South is the energy or spirit of the person and the quality of the person's will. The South is the development of the person's sexuality, of innocence and youthfulness. The colors are red and orange, and the time of life is adolescence. The lion and the wand represent the southern direction.

The East. The element is the air. The season is spring, representing new beginnings. All the senses are involved, for they seem to come alive again after the long winter months. The time is sunrise, the beginning of a new day—dawn. The color is green, and the time of life is birth and early childhood. This direction brings the power of the mind to know and understand. Illumination and the eagle represent the direction of the rising sun, along with the sword.

The West. The element is water, and the season is autumn. This direction represents courage, the courage to dare to face our deepest fears and strongest emotions. This direction is linked with our emotions. The time of day is the sunset, and the colors are blue and purple. The time of life is the adult, the time when family and career are developed. The West is linked with the creatures of the oceans and with a chalice holding wine or salt water.

An altar with objects that are precious and empowering to the mother is placed in the middle of the circle. This may consist of a bouquet of flowers; corn meal (for the washing of the feet); combs and decorations for the hair; cedar, sage (*Salvia officinalis*), and sweetgrass or whatever else may be desired for smudging. (The smudging is the burning of the previously mentioned herbs that some believe acts as a cleansing of the soul, of the aura. It is a Native American ritual, akin to the Roman Catholic Church's burning of incense during High Mass for purification purposes.) Favorite herbal teas can be brewed for a tea ceremony and placed on the altar. Special stones, jewelry, feathers, shells, seeds, gourds, and other objects of nature may be added. Fruit with seeds, eggs, crystals, and soil ready for the sowing of seeds—all can be symbolic of a woman's womb and look beautiful on the altar. Various religious and spiritual artifacts can be added to the altar, depending on one's own spiritual beliefs. Some people like to use bells, chimes, and candles. The participants can place their special objects on the altar to express their strength and well wishes. All these items can be placed on a special cloth, a baby blanket, or a shawl that the mother may use while in labor.

The participants are invited to bring offerings to the pregnant mother that are meaningful to them; examples are a poem, a drawing, a song, music, a dance, or something that has been made specifically for the pregnant mother or for the baby.

Once everyone in the circle is seated and the altar is set, the room should be silent. The pregnant mother is seated in a place of honor, preferably elevated above the rest of the group, perhaps on a cushion or a chair. Once the ceremony begins, no one is permitted to leave the circle, except for the children, because people coming and going can disturb the concentration and energy created by the group.

There are different ways to begin. I find that forming a "birth canal" and singing is a wonderful way to create the feelings of unity and support essential for every birthing mother. The "birth canal" is formed with two people holding hands and forming an arch as children do when they sing "London Bridge is Falling Down." One by one, people go through and hold hands in the same manner, contributing to a continuation of the arch. Meanwhile, the song, "From a woman we were born into this circle, from a woman we were born unto this world," is sung while people are passing through the birth canal. The participants can make up a melody for the song. The pregnant mother is the last to go through. Before each person goes through the canal, they are smudged with cedar, sage, and sweetgrass, or whatever herb is desired. The Native Americans believe that the smoke from these herbs is purifying. The dried herbs are traditionally put in an abalone shell and burned, but any fireproof shell or bowl will do. The Native Americans use a sacred eagle feather to wave the smoke over the person. Because the eagle is an endangered species, any large feather will do. I have seen crow feathers, hawk feathers, and buzzard feathers used.

After everyone is seated, bells may be rung and cymbals chimed, or a rattle may be used to focus everyone on prayer. If desired, a candle may be lit. A prayer or a song led by the midwife can be said. The prayer is sent to whatever god, goddess, or spirit the mother wishes to honor through her thanks, as well as to ask for strength and wisdom. A traditional midwife suggested the following prayer: "Thank you for the sacred circle, thank you for the woman here. We are calling together to pray for [the pregnant mother] to help her be strong through her experience and we are thanking you for all the blessings that you are giving us."

The Native American way of prayer is not to ask for anything, but to give thanks for all that one has. In many spiritual teachings, a prayer of surrender ("Thy will be done") is used. This is a very important prayer, because in nature there really are no guarantees. By saying "Thy will be done," we accept the notion that sometimes things do not happen the way we may plan. Sometimes, when nature takes its course, a water birth, a homebirth, or more rarely a vaginal birth may not happen. A prayer for a healthy mother and baby is the ultimate wish for a good outcome.

After the invocation, songs that the mother requests are sung in a lovely continuation of the ceremony. Next, a ball of yarn is passed from person to person. The yarn is wrapped around each person's wrist; it is not cut but connects all the participants. The yarn symbolizes the umbilical cord that links us all to each other and to our God. This act also symbolizes the unity of support for the pregnant mother. At the close of the circle, the yarn is cut and tied around each person's wrist as a reminder of the Blessing Way, the mother, and the good wishes to be sent to the mother and baby.

I have been to several Blessing Ways, including one that was given to me. I have found that wearing the yarn during the days or weeks following the ceremony is a wonderful reminder to send love and well wishes to the mother. When I was the pregnant mother, it reminded me of all my friends who gave me support and sent me love. Looking at the yarn gave me the combined strength of all the individuals at my ritual. The yarn is also a strong reminder when one loses faith or strength in one's self. When I looked at that yarn during my labor, I remembered the love of my friends.

After the yarn is passed, but before it is cut, the midwife calls upon the four directions, whereupon the women representing the four directions give their gifts and their well-wishes. Then the others in the circle do the same. It is important that everyone speak from the heart and put some thought into what they are giving or saying to the pregnant mother. This is a very special time, and if the well-wishes are superficial, the meaning will be lost. For some, it is a time for an outpouring of tears of love. It was so gratifying and endearing for me to hear all the good wishes from my friends during my Blessing Way, for seldom do we have the opportunity to realize how much our friends love us.

The next part of the ceremony, the footbath, simply put, is delicious. We all deserve pampering, and who deserves it more than a woman ready to go into labor? The footbath is given by the midwife to show her service to the mother. It is healing and moving to experience the care and love that is given at this time. The mother's feet and calves are washed in a large bowl filled with the tea of aromatic herbs. The herbs can be of the mother's choice and can be left in the water as well. Some suggested herbs are scented geraniums, roses, mint, comfrey, marjoram, red raspberry, grape, honeysuckle, yarrow, bay, and lavender. During the footbath, the pregnant woman's mother or mother-surrogate can be combing or brushing the pregnant woman's hair. Arranging the hair with combs or flowers or ribbons is always a treat, for few of us do this for ourselves. The changing of the hair can also be symbolic of the transition and change that the pregnant mother will go through during labor.

Songs are being sung during this time. Suggested songs are: "Oh Lord, make me strong as a bear. Yana Ohwe Ya Ho Wey Ha Ney." Another is "Open me up so I might receive, Open me up so that I might believe." "Listen, listen to my heart's song; Listen, listen to my heart's song, I will never forget you. I will never forsake you. I will always remember. I will always be true." "Dear sister, dear sister, Let me tell you how I'm feeling. You have given us your treasure. We love you so." "I am a hollow reed, open up and let the light shine through me." These and other folk songs have been handed down through the generations by oral tradition.

After the footbath, the feet and calves are rubbed and dried with blue corn meal which the Native Americans consider valuable and sacred, representing the source of life and nourishment from Mother Earth. So, drying the mother's feet with the corn meal represents giving the mother the best we have. It also helps her to draw in the nourishment and strength that she needs. At this time, reflexology points (points on the foot that some say connect with different areas of the body) can be massaged if she likes. A warm herbal tea may be given to the mother to drink and may be shared with the rest of the circle.

The pregnant mother now lies down in the middle of the circle and everyone lays hands on her, sending her strength, love, and healing. The song "May the blessings of the Goddess rest upon you" is sung.

Before everyone leaves, a sheet of paper is passed around so that people can sign up to help with meals, laundry, and cleanup for the first few weeks after the baby is born. Everyone *must* remember that when they return to perform their services, it is only to do what needs to be done and to leave, for visiting can wear out the mother and the new baby.

While working with Igor Charkowsky at the Black Sea, I saw the magnitude of the empowerment that the Blessing Way bestows. Part of the theme at the Black Sea was to exchange knowledge and ideas, as well as to birth babies in the sea. One of the women waiting to give birth was a Russian medical doctor. She was one of the more quiet members of the group and somehow did not appear to be prepared to give birth. She seemed too fragile and a bit too reserved. The other Russian women were extremely robust, self-contained, individuals, who looked like they could move boulders.

Each Blessing Way is different and takes on its own tone; the Black Sea ritual had its own unique quality as well. While performing the smudging, traditional Russian songs were sung. Some of these songs had to be sung by some of the older persons present, because the songs had been frowned upon for years. At this point I noticed the pregnant doctor whose eyes seemed to become as wide as saucers. She didn't quite know what to think or expect. She grew calm and serene as the people spoke to her in their native tongue of their good wishes and their encouragements. When it was Charkowsky's turn, he took a dolphin tee-shirt off his back that I had brought him from the states and gave it to her. This gift from Charkowsky, who is a man with few posessions, touched her deeply. After everyone encircled her and bestowed their hugs and kisses, her whole presence seemed to change. She seemed less curled inward, she sat up straighter, and she held her head up high. Her presence was now one of strength and courage, and she seemed illuminated. She then dove into the Black Sea and swam until she was nearly out of sight. Her midwife dove in after her, getting a little concerned for her welfare. After this empowerment, the doctor said she felt like she could have swum all the way to Turkey. She now felt ready to give birth, and on her return she and her husband sat down and sang traditional Russian folk songs for an hour. It was truly an awe-inspiring moment. It showed me the value of the Blessing Way and what it can do for gathering up strength. Every pregnant woman should have the opportunity to have this experience before she gives birth. I consider it one of the essentials for good prenatal care.

SUGGESTED READINGS

Airola, Paavo. *Every Woman's Book*. Phoenix: Health Plus Publishers, 1979.

Baker, Jeanine Parvati. *Conscious Conception*. Berkeley, Calif.: North Atlantic Books, 1986.

———. *Prenatal Yoga and Natural Birth*. Monroe, Utah: Freestone Publishing, 1974.

Balaskas, Janet. *New Active Birth*. London: Unwin Hyman Ltd., 1993.

Balaskas, Janet, and Gordon, Yehudi. *Water Birth*. London: Unwin Hyman Ltd., 1990.

Baldwin, Rahima. *Special Delivery*. Berkeley, Calif.: Celestial Arts, 1986.

Berends, Polly Berriens. *Whole Child/Whole Parent*. New York: Harper and Row, 1983.

Davis, Elizabeth. *Heart and Hands*. Berkeley, Calif.: Celestial Arts, 1987.

Kitzinger, Sheila. *The Complete Book of Pregnancy and Childbirth*. New York: Alfred A. Knopf, 1981.

La Leche League International. *Womanly Art of Breastfeeding*. Franklin Park, Ill.: Interstate Printers and Publishers, Inc., 1976.

Leboyer, Frederick. *Birth Without Violence*. New York: Alfred A. Knopf, 1975.

Liedloff, Jean. *The Continuum Concept*. New York: Warner Books, 1977.

Mitford, Jessica. *The American Way of Birth*. New York: Penguin Books, 1992.

Morgan, Elaine. *Descent of Woman*. New York: Stein and Day, 1972.

———. *The Aquatic Ape*. London: Souvenir Press, 1982.

Nilsson, Lennart. *A Child Is Born*. New York: Delacorte Press, 1977.

Noble, Elizabeth. *Essential Exercises for the Childbearing Year*. Boston: Houghton Mifflin Co., 1982.

Odent, Michel. *Birth Reborn*. New York: Pantheon Books, 1984.

———. *Water and Sexuality*. New York: Viking Penguin Inc., 1990.

Pearce, Joseph Chilton. *The Magical Child*. New York: E. P. Dutton, 1977.

Schwab, Michael, and Inke Schwab. *Start Well!* Minneapolis: Winston Press Inc., 1984.

Sidenbladh, Erik. *Water Babies.* New York: St. Martin's Press, 1982.

Thevenin, Tine. *The Family Bed.* P.O. Box 16004, Minneapolis, Minn. 55416.

Timmermans, Claire. *How to Teach Your Baby to Swim.* New York: Stein and Day, 1982.

Weed, Susun. *Wise Woman Herbal for the Childbearing Year.* Woodstock, N.Y.: Ash Tree Publications, 1986.

BIBLIOGRAPHY

Aderhold, Kathleen, and Perry, Leslie. "Jet Hydrotherapy for Labor and Post Partum Pain Relief." *American Journal of Maternal Child Nursing* 16 (March/April 1991).

Airola, Paavo. *Every Woman's Book.* Phoenix: Health Plus Publishers, 1979.

Baker, Jeanine Parvati. "The Dolphin Midwife." Studio City, Calif.: *Pre- and Perinatal Psychology News* 2:1 (1988).

———. *Prenatal Yoga and Natural Birth.* Monroe, Utah: Freestone Publishing, 1974.

Balaskas, Janet. *New Active Birth.* London: Unwin Hyman Paperbacks, 1993.

Balaskas, Janet, and Gordon, Yehudi. *Water Birth.* London: Unwin Hyman Ltd., 1990.

Berends, Polly Berriens. *Whole Child / Whole Parent.* New York: Harper and Row, 1983.

Boulvain, M., and Wesel, Serge. The Secretion of Endorphin, Cortisol, and Prolactin. Hospital de Frainel'alleud Waterloo, Braine l'Alleud, Belgium. Unpublished study, 1985.

Brazelton, T. B. "Observations of Neonatal Behavior: The Effects of Peri-Natal Variables in Particular That of Maternal Medication." *Journal of Child Psychiatry* 4 (1965), 613.

———. "The Remarkable Talents of the Newborn." *Birth and the Family Journal* 5:4 (Winter 1978).

Brazelton, T. B., and Robey, J. S. "Effect of Prenatal Drugs on the Behavior of the Neonate." *American Journal of Psychiatry* 126 (1970), 1261–66.

Brown, Christine. "Therapeutic Effects of Bathing During Labor." *Journal of Nurse-Midwifery* 27:1 (January/February 1982).

Butler, Simone. "Underwater Birth: A Technique or a Philosophy?" *ICEA News (International Childbirth Education Association)* 23:2 (May 1984).

Chamberlin, David. *Babies Remember Birth.* Los Angeles: Tarcher Inc., 1988.

Church, Linda. "Waterbirth: One Birthing Center's Observations." *Journal of Nurse-Midwifery* 34:4 (July/August 1989).

Clarke, Pat. "Water Birth." *Midwives Chronicle and Nursing Notes* (July 1989).

Coghill, Rona. "To the Water Born." *Nursing Times* 88:24 (June 10, 1992).

Cohen, Nancy Wainer, and Estner, Lois J. *Silent Knife.* South Hadley, Mass.: Bergin and Garvey, 1983.

Coletti, L. "Relationship Between Pregnancy and Birth Complications and Later Development of Learning Disabilities." *Journal of Learning Disabilities* 12 (1979), 25–29.

Croutier, Alev. *Taking the Waters.* New York: Abbeville Press, 1992.

DeliQuadri, Lyn, and Breckenridge, Kati. *The New Mother Care.* Boston: Tarcher, 1978.

De Smidt, Leon Sylvester. *Among the San Blas Indians of Panama.* Troy, N.Y.: HRAF 844 Cuna. (1948).

Emerson, Sally. *A Celebration of Babies.* London: Blackie and Son Ltd., 1986.

Engelmann, George J. *Labor Among Primitive Peoples.* St. Louis: J. H. Chambers and Co. 1882.

Faber, Adele, and Mazlish, Elaine. *How to Talk So Kids Will Listen and Listen So Kids Will Talk.* New York: Avon, 1980.

Ford, Linda, and Garland, Dianne. "An Aqua Birth Concept." *Midwives Chronicle and Nursing Notes* (July 1989).

Ford Heritage. *Composition and Facts About Foods.* Health Research, Box 70 Mokelumne Hill, Calif. 95245. 1971.

Frye, Anne. *Understanding Lab Work in the Childbearing Year.* New Haven, Conn.: Labrys Press, 1990.

Garrey, Matthew, et al. *Obstetrics Illustrated.* 2d ed. New York: Churchill Livingstone, 1974.

Gordon, Thomas. *Parent Effectiveness Training.* New York: New American Library, 1975.

Greenberg, Martin, and Morris, Norman. "Engrossment: The Newborn's Impact upon the Father." *American Journal of Orthopsychiatry* 4:44 (July 1974).

Greenleaf, John. Physiological Responses to Prolonged Bed Rest and Fluid Immersion In Humans. Laboratory for Human Environmental Physiology, Biomedical Division, NASA-Ames Research Center, Moffett Field, Calif. 94035 (1984).

Guyton, Arthur. *Textbook of Medical Physiology.* 5th ed. Philadelphia: W. B. Saunders Co., 1976.

Haire, Doris. Testimony before the California Commission on Crime Control and Violence Prevention, San Francisco, September 1980.

Hansen, K., Hofmeyr, G. J., and Silcock, L. "Birth Under Water." Johannesburg Hospital and University of the Witwaterstand, South Africa. Unpublished paper.

Hardy, Sir Alister. "Was Man More Aquatic In the Past?" *The New Scientist,* 1960.

Harlow, H. F., and Means, Clara. *The Human Model: Primate Perspectives.* (Washington, D.C.: Winston and Sons, 1978).

Hellman, Louis, et al. *Williams Obstetrics.* 14th ed. New York: Appleton-Century-Crofts, 1971.

Homer, Nils, and Wassen, Henry. *Mu-Igala or the Way of Muu: A Medicine Song from the Cuna Indians of Panama.* Goteborg: HRAF 844 Cuna. (1947).

Hunter, R. S., et al. "Antecedents of Child Abuse and Neglect in Premature Infants: A Prospective Study in a Newborn Intensive Care Unit." *Pediatrics* 61 (1978), 629.

Iglesias, Marvel Elya, and Morgan, Christine. *From the Cradle to the Grave.* Cristobol: HRAF 844 Cuna. (1939).

Johnson, Buffie. *Lady of the Beasts.* San Francisco: Harper and Row Inc., 1988.

Jones, Sandy. "Michel Odent." *Mothering Magazine* (Fall 1983).

Jones, Wood. *Man's Place Among the Mammals.* London: Arnold and Co., 1929.

Katz, Vern, et al. "Fetal and Uterine Responses to Immersion and Exercise." *Obstetrics and Gynecology* 72:2 (1988).

Kay, Margarita. *Anthropology of Human Birth.* Philadelphia: F. A. Davis Co., 1982.

Kitzinger, Sheila. "Sheila Kitzinger's Letter from England." *Birth* 18:3 (1991).

Klaus, Marshall H., and Kennell, J. *Maternal Infant Bonding.* St. Louis: Mosley, 1976).

Klein, Michael. "Birth Room Transfer and Procedure Rates—What Do They Tell About the Setting?" *Birth* 10:2 (1983).

Kroska, Rita, and Carroll, Mary. "Use of Water in Labor." *Birth* 9:1 (1982), 47.

Lagercrantz, Hugo, and Slotkin, Theodore A. "The Stress of Being Born." *Scientific American* (April 1986).

Leatherwood, Stephen, and Reeves, Randall R. *The Sierra Club Handbook of Whales and Dolphins.* San Francisco: Sierra Club Books, 1979.

Lebherz, Thomas B., et al. "Premature Rupture of Membranes." *American Journal of OB. Gyn* 81 (1960), 658–665.

Leboyer, Frederick. *Birth Without Violence.* New York: Alfred A. Knopf, 1975.

Leonard, Jim, and Laut, Phil. *Rebirthing: The Science of Enjoying All of Your Life.* Hollywood: Trinity Publications, 1983.

Levinson, Gershon, and Shnider, Sol M. "Catecholamines: The Effects of Maternal Fear and Its Treatment on Uterine Function and Circulation." *Birth and the Family Journal* 6:3 (Fall 1979).

Levkoff, Abner. "Fetal Adaptation to Extrauterine Life." *Maternal Fetal Medicine: Principles of Practice.* Philadelphia: W. B. Saunders Co., 1982.

Liedloff, Jean. *The Continuum Concept.* New York: Warner Books, 1977.

Lockley, Ronald M. *Whales, Dolphins, and Porpoises.* Methuen of Australia: PTY LTD, 1979.

Marshall, Donald. *Cuna Folk.* Unpublished Manuscript. Cambridge, Mass.: Harvard University, HRAF 844 Cuna. (1950).

Milner, Isobel. "Water Birth for Pain Relief in Labour." *Nursing Times* 84:1 (January 6, 1988).

Morgan, Elaine. *The Descent of Woman.* New York: Stein and Day, 1972.

———. *The Aquatic Ape.* London: Souvenir Press, 1982.

Myles, Margaret. *Textbook for Midwives.* 8th ed. New York: Churchill Livingstone, 1975.

Newton, Carol. "Bath Rights." *Nursing Times* 88:24 (June 10, 1992).

Nilsson, Lennart. *A Child Is Born*. New York: Delacorte Press, 1977.

Noble, Elizabeth. *Essential Exercises for the Childbearing Year*. Boston: Houghton Mifflin Co., 1982.

Norris, Kenneth. *Whales, Dolphins, and Porpoises*. Berkeley: University of California Press, 1966.

O'Connor, S., et al. "Reduced Incidence of Parenting Inadequacy Following Rooming-In." *Pediatrics* 66 (1980), 176–82.

Odent, Michel. "Birth Under Water." *The Lancet* 24/31 (December 1983).

———. *Birth Reborn*. New York: Pantheon Books, 1984.

———. "The Evolution of Obstetrics at Pithiviers." *Birth and the Family Journal* 8:1 (1981).

O'Hare, J. P., et al. "Observations on the Effects of Immersion in Bath Spa Water." *British Medical Journal* 291 (December 1985).

Pagana, Kathleen, and Pagana, Timothy. *Mosby's Diagnostic and Laboratory Test Reference*. St. Louis, Mo.: Mosby, 1992.

Porter, Barbara. "Water Births: The Pros—and Cons." *ICEA NEWS* 23:3 (August 1984), 3–4.

Rice, Ruth. "Infant Stress and the Relationship to Violent Behavior." *The Journal of Neonatal Nursing* 3:5 (April 1985).

Roth, Tovert. Testimony before the California Commission on Crime Control and Violence Prevention, San Francisco, September 1980.

Sagov, Stanley, et al. *Home Birth, A Practitioner's Guide to Birth Outside the Hospital*. Rockville, Md.: Aspen Publications, 1984.

Schwenk, Theodor. *Sensitive Chaos, The Creation of Flowing Forms in Water and Air*. New York: Schocken Books, 1976.

Schwenk, Theodor, and Schwenk, Wolfram. *Water: The Element of Life*. Hudson, N.Y.: Anthroposophic Press Inc., 1989.

Sibley, L., et al. "Swimming and Physical Fitness During Pregnancy." *Journal of Nurse-Midwifery* 26:6 (1981).

Sidenbladh, Erik. *Water Babies*. New York: St. Martin's Press, 1982.

Smith, Myra. Effect of Warm Tub Bathing During Labor. Unpublished abstract, Grady Memorial Hospital, Atlanta, Georgia, 1987.

Stout, David. *Handbook of South American Indians*. Washington, D.C.: Government Printing Office, HRAF 844 Cuna. (1948).

———. *San Blas Cuna Acculturation*. New York: Viking Fund, HRAF 844 Cuna. (1947).

Tew, Marjorie. *Safer Childbirth?* New York: Chapman Hall, 1990.

Thevenin, Tine. *The Family Bed*. P.O. Box 16004, Minneapolis, Minn. 55416.

Timmermans, Claire. *How to Teach Your Baby to Swim*. New York: Stein & Day, 1975.

Trevathan, Wenda R. *Human Birth: An Evolutionary Perspective*. New York: Aldine De Gruyter, 1987.

Varney, Helen. *Nurse-Midwifery*. Boston: Blackwell Scientific Publications, 1987.

Verney, Thomas. *The Secret Life of the Unborn Child*. New York: Summit Books, 1981.

Waldenstrom, Ulla, and Nilsson, Carl-Axel. "Warm Tub Bath After Sponta-
    neous Rupture of the Membranes." *Birth* 19:2 (June 1992).
Wertz, Richard, and Wertz, Dorthy. *Lying In.* New York: Free Press, 1977.
White, Gregory. *Emergency Childbirth: A Manual.* Police Train.: n.d.
Zimmerman, R. "Water Birth—Is It Safe?" *Journal of Perinatal Medicine* 21:1
    (1993).

INDEX

About the Author

SUSANNA NAPIERALA is a certified midwife and home birth attendant in the State of California. She has trained worldwide in the methods of water birth and has served as an advisor for the World Health
Organization.